Fathers and family centres
Engaging fathers in preventive services

Deborah Ghate, Catherine Shaw and Neal Hazel

The **Joseph Rowntree Foundation** has supported this project as part of its programme of research and innovative development projects, which it hopes will be of value to policy makers and practitioners. The facts presented and views expressed in this report are, however, those of the authors and not necessarily those of the Foundation.

POLICY ● RESEARCH BUREAU

The Policy Research Bureau is an independent, not-for-profit, social policy research unit specialising in research on children, young people and families.

© Joseph Rowntree Foundation 2000

All rights reserved.

Published for the Joseph Rowntree Foundation by YPS

ISBN 1 902633 49 0

Prepared and printed by:
York Publishing Services Ltd
64 Hallfield Road
Layerthorpe
York YO31 7ZQ
Tel: 01904 430033; Fax: 01904 430868; E-mail: orders@yps,ymn.co.uk

Contents

		Page
Acknowledgements		iv
1	**Introduction and background to the study**	1
	What is a family centre?	1
	Why offer support to fathers?	1
	Objectives of the study	2
2	**Methodology**	4
	Stage 1 – selecting local authorities and, within them, family centres	4
	Stage 2 – selecting a sample of individuals	6
	Social and ethnic profile of interviewees	8
	Data collection and analysis	8
3	**Barriers to men's use of family centres**	10
	Introduction	10
	Barriers at the family centre level	11
4	**Enabling factors in men's use of family centres**	29
	Introduction	29
	Enabling factors at the family centre level	30
5	**Conclusions and implications for policy and practice**	43
	Who are family centres for? – 'child-focused' versus 'family-focused' services	43
	The need for clarity of focus	45
	Making family centres father-friendly: possible directions for change in policy and practice	46
References		50
Appendix 1: Practice issues in engaging with fathers in family centres		51
Appendix 2: Range of activities taking place in sample family centres		52
Appendix 3: Pen portraits of family centres		53

Acknowledgments

We gratefully acknowledge the financial support of the Joseph Rowntree Foundation throughout this project and the advice and help of Susan Taylor, Senior Research Manager at the Foundation, who oversaw the project.

The Joseph Rowntree Foundation convened an Advisory Group for the study, who met with us three times during the course of the project and provided valuable advice, feedback, suggestions and encouragement. Members of the Advisory Group were: Jabeer Butt, REU (formerly Race Equality Unit); Naomi Eisenstadt, then Chief Executive, Family Service Units; Trefor Lloyd, Working with Men; Teresa Smith, Head of the Department of Applied Social Studies and Social Research at the University of Oxford; Professor Jane Tunstill, Royal Holloway University of London; Ian Vallender, Family Centres Network and National Council for Voluntary Child Care Organisation (NCVCCO); and Peter Welply, Manager, Cuddesden Corner Family Centre, Oxford.

Other organisations which were generous with help and advice include: numerous local authority Social Services Departments; the Ormiston Trust; NCH Action for Children; The Children's Society; Barnardo's; the NSPCC; Spurgeon's Child Care; Children in Wales; Children in Scotland; Children North East; Fathers Plus; the Family Support Network at University of East Anglia; and the Family Centre Network at NCVCCO. We would also like to thank Kate Oakley who carried out some of the fieldwork.

We would like to extend our warmest thanks to the family centres which took part, although we have not named them for reasons of confidentiality. We were extremely fortunate in the time, help and support we received from centre managers and staff, who were unfailingly kind and tolerant of our disruption to their daily routine, ferried us to remote interviews and kept us supplied with cups of tea throughout. Last but not least, we would like to express our appreciation to the families who took part in the study, many of whom allowed us into their homes and were generous with time and information.

The interpretations and opinions expressed in this report are those of the Policy Research Bureau alone and we are, of course, solely responsible for any errors or mistakes.

1 Introduction and background to the study

In 1997 the Joseph Rowntree Foundation (JRF) invited research proposals as part of a new research and development initiative, designed to promote the development of 'effective mainstream support to prevent family breakdown'. This report describes a qualitative study carried out in 1998–99 as part of this initiative by the Policy Research Bureau. The study explored barriers and enabling factors in the participation and engagement with preventative services of one of the JRF's key interest groups – fathers (including biological fathers, step-fathers and partners of women with children). In particular, the study focused on fathers' engagement with one important aspect of mainstream family support services – family centres.

The study was large and complex, focusing not only on issues connected with family centres themselves, but also on background contextual factors in families' lives that influence the need for – and use of – family support services more generally. However, this report is intended primarily for policy and practice audiences, and thus presents only the key findings of direct relevance to practice. Although social, cultural and individual-level factors are important for understanding the context against which family centres are setting out to attract fathers, the research suggested that issues connected with the way family centres are structured and run were more significant for understanding why men do, or don't, use these services. Furthermore, factors operating at the family-centre level are, of course, the most amenable to change at the policy and practice level, and present the greatest opportunity in terms of developing models for father-friendly services.

The research is discussed in its wider context, together with further data, additional findings and fuller background, methodological and technical information, in Ghate *et al.* (2000).

What is a family centre?

Family centres (also sometimes referred to as 'family projects' or 'children's centres') are a well-established, community-based component of family-support provision. Indeed, it would not be overstating the case to say that they occupy a central position in the wider matrix of service for families and children across the UK. Family centres vary greatly in ethos, structure, organisational culture and the activities in which they engage. They also vary in size, location, resourcing, staffing and user profile. They frequently offer both primary and secondary prevention services to families within their local catchment areas (Pugh *et al.*, 1994), providing open access services aimed at parents and children within the wider community, as well as referral-based services that are targeted more specifically at families with children 'in need' or thought to be 'at risk' of various forms of child abuse and neglect (Children Act 1989). As such, family centres can be seen as being on the front-line of mainstream preventive services for families in the UK.

Why offer support to fathers?

There is now growing research evidence that promoting and encouraging fathers' greater involvement in child-care can enhance outcomes for children, especially in terms of psycho-social development (Kraemer, 1995; Lamb, 1996). On both sides of the Atlantic and across Europe, fatherhood is increasingly emerging as a key issue in both family policy and family support practice (Levine and Pitt 1995; Burghes et al. 1997). In the UK, 'Fatherhood [is] on the agenda as never before' (Burgess and Ruxton, 1996).

Yet, in spite of increasing policy and practice interest in fatherhood, provision of services for men as child-carers lags behind that for women. Fathers are neither well-served by generic 'family support' services, nor are they widely catered for as parents in their own right. Family centres are no exception to this. Amongst all the work that has been done on profiling users of family centres (whether open-access users or referred users), one fact stands out with great clarity: fathers have been largely absent – both physically and conceptually – from the picture. Yet family centres, at least in principle, offer an ideal opportunity to help fathers become more involved and more competent in child-care, and most parents and family centre staff who took part in this study would agree that supporting fathers is a worthwhile endeavour. Most were convinced of the likely benefits of this for children, women and for men themselves.

In summary, the absence of men from family support services and the need to make services more accessible and acceptable to fathers has become an area of growing concern for policy-makers and practitioners alike. Failure to engage fathers in the work of family centres and the lack of research into the underlying reasons for this failure, have real consequences for the extent to which centres can work effectively with parents of both sexes and their children. Given our increasing awareness of the potential benefits of fathers' greater involvement in child-care, this must be seen as a missed opportunity at both the primary and secondary prevention levels. Ultimately, we hoped that the findings from this research would enable us to provide concrete recommendations for improving this situation. We wanted to highlight ways in which family centres can be made more accessible and acceptable to fathers, as well as to mothers, whilst acknowledging the possible implications of this for family centres as they currently exist.

Objectives of the study

The study set out to explore possible explanations for fathers' relative lack of involvement with family centres from the multiple perspectives of:

- men already using family centres (both married/partnered and lone fathers), whom we term 'involved'

- men not using centres (but with partners who were involved with the centre), whom we term 'uninvolved'

- the wives and partners of these men

- staff and managers in family centres.

The study was unusual in including not only the perceptions of men using family centres (which is rare), but also the views of men *not* using centres. To our knowledge, no other studies have yet taken this approach. We included women's perspectives because they are the dominant existing 'clientele' of family centres and perhaps stand to lose, as well as to gain, from attempts to widen the client base to include more fathers. Our principal aim was to explore the barriers and enabling factors in

Introduction and background to the study

fathers' use of family centres.

In thinking about the concept of involvement, we considered both 'entry-level' involvement (men being on the premises) and 'engagement' at a deeper level (men actually participating in family centre activities). More specifically, we hoped to find out:

- How do men who are not involved with family centres view the centres? Why do they not attend? What puts them off or prevents them from becoming more involved? What, if anything, would encourage them to get more involved?

- What are the experiences of men who are involved with centres? What do they do there? What do they get out of attending and do they get what they want? How could centres be improved to attract more men?

- What are the perspectives of women and staff? Do they want men to use the centre? What do they see as the benefits and disadvantages of having men around in family centres? Why do they think men do or don't use the centre? Do they see scope for change, or greater engagement with fathers?

2 Methodology

As befits a relatively new area of research, we used mainly qualitative (unstructured) methods to gather and analyse the data for this study. A small-scale, detailed, exploratory study of this type was more suited to our aims than a broader-brush but more superficial survey of a larger number of fathers and family centres.

The sample for the study was drawn in two main stages. Stage one involved drawing a sample of local authorities and subsequently of family centres, while stage two involved recruiting a sample of individuals associated with those centres.

Stage 1 – selecting local authorities and, within them, family centres

Our aim was to recruit a sample of family centres that represented, as far as is possible, the range and diversity of centres. To do this we selected seven local authorities across England and Wales[1] to achieve a cross-section of service provision contexts, taking into account region, whether urban or rural population, and the type of authority. We then audited family centre provision in each location, collating information from a range of sources to compile a complete list of centres within the authority.

Having compiled what we believed to be a reasonably comprehensive list of all family centres in each authority, we then conducted a telephone survey to gather basic classificatory information about each centre on our list. This information is shown in Box 1.

> **Box 1 Classificatory information collected as part of the audit of family centres**
>
> - Type of community served (urban, rural, in need/at risk or wider community)
>
> - Type of work mainly carried out:
>   A social work/child protection
>   B neighbourhood/community-based
>   C community development
>   D service/day-care/early years/ nursery/community child-care
>   E mixture of above
>
> - Source of funding [local authority (LA), voluntary or partnership]
>
> - Management/accountability (LA, voluntary, partnership)
>
> - Number of service users
>
> - Staffing
>
> - Range of activities
>
> - Numbers of fathers using the centre, if any, and status (lone or partnered)
>
> - Whether special designated activities for fathers
>
> - Priority attached to/level of need perceived regarding work with fathers

After the audit, we selected two centres in each authority, aiming to achieve, in the sample as a whole, a spread of characteristics as shown in Box 2.

Methodology

> **Box 2 Spread of characteristics sought in sampled family centres**
>
> **Management/funding**
> - statutory sector
> - voluntary sector
> - statutory/voluntary partnership
>
> **Typology**
> - range of types A–E
> - referred cases and 'heavy-end' child protection
> - assessment and court reports
> - open-access, drop-in facilities
>
> **Work with fathers**
> - working with fathers a priority
> - working with fathers not a priority
>
> **Size**
> - large
> - small
>
> **Range of activities**
> - wide
> - narrow

Each centre was contacted individually and invited to participate in the study. Of the 14 centres approached, only one was unable to take part. Thus 13 centres from seven local authorities formed the final sample of family centres.

The sample included examples of all the 'types' of family centre described above and covered a broad range of different funding and management arrangements, as shown in Table 1.

The six local authority centres were all run either by social services or early-years departments. Even within this group we found a range of different policy and practice contexts. Some centres were one of several run by the authority, each providing a more or less identical set of services to its particular catchment area, often based around child protection and assessment work. By contrast, in other authorities, centre managers had been allowed considerable autonomy in developing their own specialised services.

The wide variety of voluntary sector family centre provision has also been reflected within our sample. We included centres which came under the umbrella of smaller local or regionally based charitable organisations, as well as those run by large national children's charities. Two of our sample centres were voluntary organisations in their own right, overseen by management committees and funded from a variety of sources. Several of these voluntary

Table 1 Sample of family centres by type of centre

Type of centre (primary function)	Local authority	Voluntary sector	Partnership	Total
A: child protection, social work	2	1	0	3
B: neighbourhood-based, open access	0	2	1	3
C: community development model	0	1	0	1
D: day-care, nursery, early years	1	0	0	1
E: mixture of two or more of the above	3	0	2	5
Total	6	4	3	13

sector centres took referrals from social services and other agencies, although only one conducted statutory assessments.

'Partnership' centres were all located within the voluntary sector, but in addition had either posts funded directly by the LA, or some LA representation on their management committee.

The centres also varied considerably in terms of size and scale. One type A centre (child protection), for example, working with up to a dozen referred families at a time, was staffed by a part-time manager supported only by sessional and voluntary workers, whilst another employed a full-time multi-disciplinary team for a similar case-load. By contrast, type B centres (neighbourhood) – all of which were located within the voluntary sector – tended to number their adult and child 'users' in hundreds over the course of a year, although the level of contact with many individuals was minimal.

In terms of premises and equipment, two centres functioned from a couple of rooms within larger organisations; a number were working from adapted or converted premises; and others were using purpose-built premises. In each case, varying degrees of investment were evident in terms of equipment and resources. We also encountered a wide range of different types of activity and service offered by the centres, which are presented in Appendix 2.

In summary, the primary feature of this sample of family centres is, perhaps, its very diversity. This is further illustrated in the brief 'pen-portraits' of the centres which are presented in Appendix 3. All centre names have been changed.

Stage 2 – selecting a sample of individuals

Our primary interest was in gaining a broad overview of the family centres in the sample, rather than in conducting a highly detailed exploration of individual centres' work. We were also concerned to keep the burden on participating centres as light as possible. We therefore designed a sampling strategy that recruited relatively few respondents from each centre, but which built up to a substantial sample overall. We asked each participating centre to help us contact:

- a couple, where the centre was working with both parents
- a couple, where the centre was working with the mother, but not the father
- any lone fathers who were using the centre in their own right
- a staff member involved in working directly with the fathers and mothers we interviewed.

Overall, the sampling strategy was designed to enable us to 'triangulate' data, i.e. to interview matched 'sets' of respondents in order to explore the key issues from multiple but related perspectives. At most centres we were successful in obtaining at least seven interviews with various combinations of respondents. These included fathers who had little or no contact with the centres used by their partners and children ('uninvolved' fathers), as well as those who took a more active part ('involved' fathers).

'Uninvolved' fathers and their partners

Thirteen interviews were conducted with men who had virtually no contact with the family

Methodology

centre, despite the involvement of their partner. The partners of these men were also interviewed.

'Involved' fathers and their partners (where applicable)

We deliberately sought out men who were either lone parents or main carers and who were therefore using the family centre 'in their own right' ($n = 15$). Three centres ran fathers' groups, and eight of the men interviewed were involved in such a group. Other 'involved' fathers were either attending the centre as part of a family referral, or on a voluntary basis alongside their partner. Interviews were also conducted with partners of most of these 'involved' fathers.[2] Altogether 15 of the 'involved' fathers interviewed were voluntary users of centre services, whereas 12 had been referred.

Staff

We also interviewed a member of staff who worked closely with each individual or family. Staff interviewed covered a wide spectrum of experience and responsibility, ranging from centre managers, teachers and social workers to unqualified play-leaders and family-support workers. Five of the staff interviewed were

Figure 1 The meaning of 'involved' and 'uninvolved': characteristics and numbers of interviewees

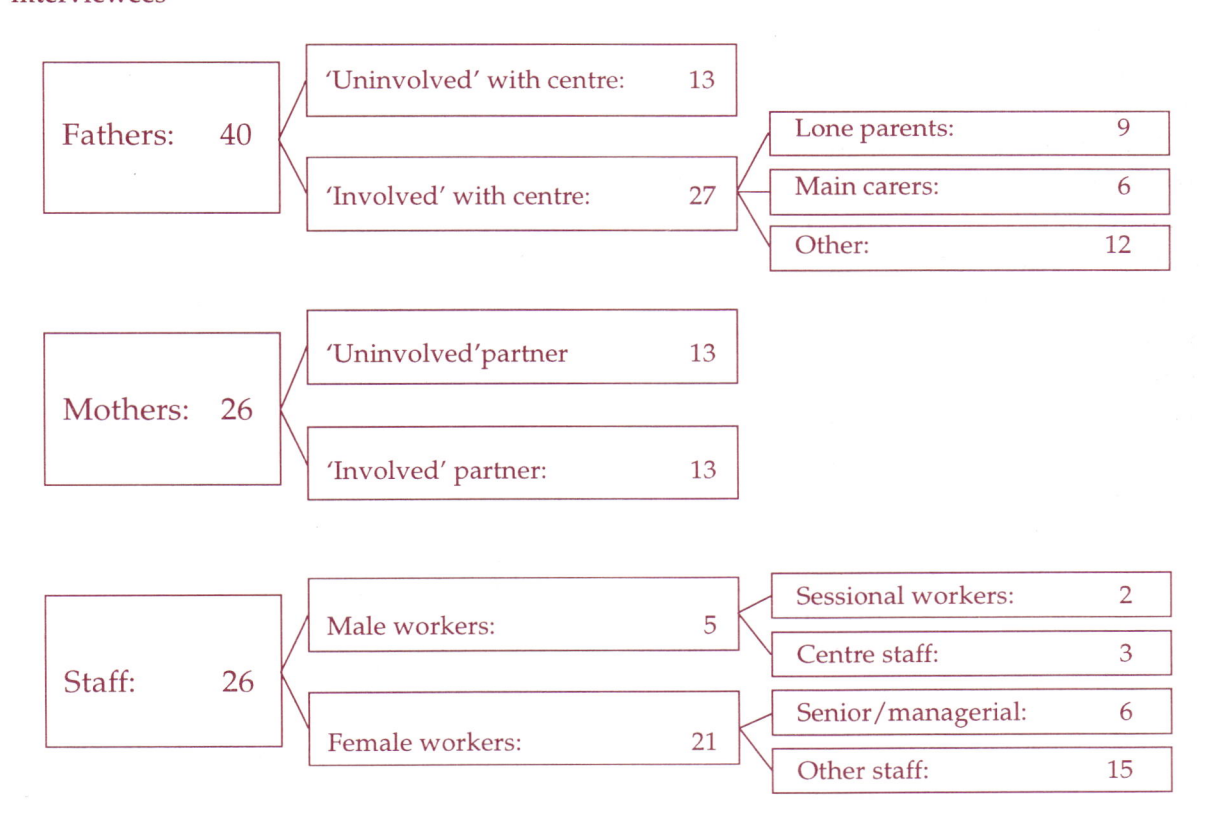

Fathers: 40
- 'Uninvolved' with centre: 13
- 'Involved' with centre: 27
  - Lone parents: 9
  - Main carers: 6
  - Other: 12

Mothers: 26
- 'Uninvolved' partner: 13
- 'Involved' partner: 13

Staff: 26
- Male workers: 5
  - Sessional workers: 2
  - Centre staff: 3
- Female workers: 21
  - Senior/managerial: 6
  - Other staff: 15

male, two of whom were employed on a sessional basis to work exclusively with fathers' groups and were not involved with other aspects of centre life.

Thus, a total of 92 individuals were interviewed in the 13 centres: 40 fathers,[3] 26 mothers and 26 members of staff. Figure 1 shows the sample of interviewees broken down further in terms of relevant characteristics.

It should be noted that the meanings of the terms 'involved' and 'uninvolved' are both relative and context-dependent, varying according to the type of centre and the range of activities on offer. At some type B (neighbourhood) or type D (day-care) centres, being 'involved' could mean little more than being the parent who picked-up or dropped-off children at the nursery each day, or perhaps an occasional drop-in user.

At the other end of the scale 'involvement' with a type A (child protection) centre could entail a commitment to attending the centre several times a week, for intensive individual family sessions over a substantial period. At centres where all cases were referred (and the 'client' was the family, as opposed to an individual), the term 'uninvolved' is clearly less appropriate, as work did not take place unless the entire family unit was engaged in the process. At such centres we attempted to ensure, by consultation with staff, that our sample included families where the father appeared to be less than optimally engaged with the work, or comfortable within the family centre setting, as well as those who could truly be described as 'involved'.

Social and ethnic profile of interviewees

Whilst most of the centres served materially disadvantaged and relatively homogenous populations, a few were located in areas having a wider social or ethnic mix. Where present, this diversity has been reflected in the profile of interviewees. Thus, while the majority of mothers and fathers interviewed had relatively little formal education or skills, a small number of interviewees were graduates, or had a professional background.

Similarly, because of the particular locations of the centres in the study, most of the interviewees were white. However, a total of eight parents interviewed (at four different centres) were from minority ethnic groups: four fathers (two involved, two uninvolved) and four mothers. We also interviewed two workers from minority ethnic groups. Even within this small number, a range of contrasting cultural backgrounds were represented: African, Caribbean, South Asian, Middle Eastern and mixed race. This diversity, taken together with the small total number involved, meant that it would not be methodologically sound for us to attempt to draw general conclusions about the experiences of interviewees from minority ethnic groups. See Ghate *et al.* (2000) for a further discussion.

Data collection and analysis

Interviews were carried out by a team of four researchers from the Bureau, either in private rooms within family centres, or in respondents' own homes. To preserve confidentiality, all interviews were carried out separately. Interviews ranged in length from 45 minutes to approximately two hours, with the average

Methodology

length being around one hour. All interviews were taped (with respondents' permission) and transcribed verbatim.

In keeping with the tradition of qualitative research as mainly inductive (i.e. conclusions are allowed to arise out of the data), analysis followed a grounded theory approach (Glaser and Straus, 1967). Grounded theory stresses the importance of staying close to the data, so that the analysis is 'grounded' in the actual words and language of the informants. Hence, in our presentation of the findings we have drawn heavily on the verbatim interview transcripts. The 'framework' technique was used to structure the analysis (Ritchie and Spencer, 1994) enabling interview data to be rigorously reviewed and categorised under thematic headings. We used WinMax, a computer-assisted qualitative data analysis software package (Kuckartz, 1998) to help sort the data before entering onto thematic charts.

Finally, during the course of drafting the report we sought feedback from our Advisory Group, other researchers and from the family centres who took part in the study. Whilst the conclusions we have drawn are, of course, entirely our own, it was reassuring to find that centres which had participated in the research felt that the findings 'chimed' with their own experiences.

Notes

1. After discussion with Scottish child-care organisations, Scotland was ruled out of the study because of its different child-care policy and practice context.
2. It was not possible or appropriate to interview the partner of every 'involved' father. In one case, where the father was the main carer, the mother had no involvement with the centre at all. At Brownfield, it was not possible to interview the partners of the men's group interviewees. Lone parents, by definition, had no partner to interview.
3. Includes a group interview with four fathers from Brownfield men's group.

3 Barriers to men's use of family centres

Introduction

As we indicated earlier, in much of the previous work that has been done on profiling users of family centres, fathers have been largely absent – both physically and conceptually – from the picture. In conducting our research into the reasons why fathers were not more fully engaged with family centre services, we investigated barriers (and enabling) factors operating at three levels:

- the broader social and cultural level
- the level of the individual
- the level of the family centre itself.

Whilst the findings presented in this report focus on those factors most amenable to change by practitioners and policy-makers (i.e. barriers and enabling factors operating at the family centre level), it would be naïve to completely overlook either the broader context in which family centres operate, or the unique circumstances and motivations of actual and potential users of their services. A brief summary of these factors and the influence they can have on fathers' engagement with family centres is presented below and discussed in further detail in Ghate *et al.* (2000). However, most of the remainder of this report focuses on findings relating to barriers operating at the family centre level.

The social and cultural context

No discussion of men's use of family support services would be complete without reference to the highly gendered nature of child-care in contemporary Britain. Despite mounting (though often anecdotal) evidence that fathers are playing an increasingly large part in child-rearing at home (see Burghes *et al.*, 1997 for a discussion) and indications that the expectations of both mothers and fathers are changing in this respect, social attitudes to fathers' involvement in child-care continue to cast the paternal role as secondary to that of mothers. By and large, child-care continues to be seen by many as 'women's work' and institutions and services frequently act to reinforce this perception. Our study uncovered many instances of such attitudes, expressed by fathers, mothers and family-centre staff.

Secondly, whilst attitudes to male roles and masculinity more generally are under scrutiny in contemporary British society, it is hardly controversial to point out that 'traditional' attitudes to masculinity persist, amongst other things emphasising self-sufficiency and independence rather than help-seeking and service-use. We came across a few interviewees (again including mothers, fathers and staff) who expressed such views (Ghate *et al.*, 2000), including a number of fathers who reported (or were reported by partners as having) negative views about family-support services in general as 'interfering'. Nevertheless, we did not find this in itself to be an insuperable barrier to fathers' involvement in family centres.

Individual circumstances and motivations

Irrespective of any barriers identifiable at the broad social and cultural level, in terms of attitudes to child-care and to family centres themselves, personal and family circumstances and other individual-level factors can also operate as a discouragement to fathers becoming involved with family-centre activities.

Practical difficulties in accessing centres were an issue for a few men, in particular

Barriers to men's use of family centres

working hours and not being able to get to centres during day-time opening hours. Of course, it could be said that opening hours are an issue of general accessibility (that is, a barrier at the centre or institutional level), rather than a problem for individual men. However, for the men in our sample, on the whole, accessibility was not as great a barrier as might have been expected as relatively few men who we interviewed were in work, or held out much expectation of finding work in the foreseeable future. Thus, at least as far as the centres in our sample were concerned, it would not be true to say that the lack of late or weekend opening hours was a major problem for many actual or potential male users.

Relationships with partners could also operate as individual-level barriers to family centre involvement. For example, sometimes wives and girlfriends made it clear they preferred not to have their partner present at the centre. Most often, though, it was the reverse circumstance – a father wanting to have time away from the family, rather than time with them – that seemed to mediate men's use of family centres. They felt there was a need to have a break from partners and children every now and again for the benefit of all concerned. Thus, as some men expressed it, sometimes the need was for men positively not to go to the centre, rather than to go.

A small minority of men seemed unlikely to be enabled or persuaded to make use of family centres, no matter what changes might take place within society as a whole or within individual centres. Some, for example, expressed (or were described as having) a total lack of interest in doing things with the family, whilst others claimed to feel so shy and self-conscious in public that use of any communal service was an ordeal. It was, however, sometimes difficult to establish the extent to which such attitudes were influenced by wider social attitudes to men and child-care, or to men and services.

Barriers at the family centre level

Barriers to fathers' use of centres located at the socio-cultural level, or at the individual and family level, may be relatively difficult to address. However, at the level of family centres themselves we hoped to identify barriers which might, at least in principle, be more amenable to change.

A major finding was that family centre 'type' did not seem to account for the variations which we found in family centre level barriers to men's greater engagement. This is perhaps not surprising, given the great variation in family-centre shape and form noted in Chapter 1. Moreover, not only did we find that there was no close association between male user involvement and broad type of centre, we also found that even *within* individual family centres, patterns were hard to discern. Often, for example, parts of the service were reaching men and parts were not; some male users felt comfortable and involved in the centre and others did not; and, frequently, staff perceptions of whether or not they were successfully working with men did not entirely 'fit' with user and non-user perceptions.

However, we did identify one factor operating at the centre level which appeared to have a definite influence on the strength of the barriers that were reported in relation to engaging fathers. This is best described as an

Fathers and family centres

overall orientation, or a broad approach to working with men. Broadly speaking we were able to group centres (or components of centres) on the basis of three broad 'orientations'. These were fundamentally defined by attitudes to working with men on the part of both staff and users, as well as by centre priorities as reflected in provision of particular services and activities. That is, our concept of 'orientation' reflected centres' approach to working with men, both in terms of how men were viewed and treated, and what provision, if any, was made for fathers using the centre.

The three overall 'orientation' groupings we identified were: gender-blind, gender-differentiated and agnostic.

The gender-blind approach

'Gender-blind' centres regarded men as the 'same' as women users. These centres tended to take the view that men should be treated exactly the same as women users, sometimes expressed in terms of an explicit policy of 'equal opportunities' within the centre.

Case example

A number of men were using these centres, sometimes with partners, sometimes alone. Activities were open to all – i.e. there were no closed, single-sex groups and the ethos was on everyone joining in together. There were some male staff, but in general no explicit attempt was made to match staff to users on the basis of sex. Staff sometimes described the approach as being underpinned by a desire to cross gender barriers and break down gender stereotypes.

For example, one centre worker said of her gender-blind centre:

We don't do men's groups, and we don't do women's groups. We don't separate them. Whatever groups we do, we run as equal, really. Everybody's welcome to that and if they don't come, that's their own choice.

The gender-differentiated approach

'Gender-differentiated' centres regarded men as different from women users. Centres of this type tended to take the view that working with men presented different challenges to working with women and both staff and users expressed views that stressed gender differences.

Case example

These centres tended to be numerically dominated by female users, but were actively trying to accommodate male users. They often hosted single-sex activities (e.g. men's groups and women-only sessions), or were trying to develop such services. In general, there was not much mixing of the sexes and fathers, where they were encountered, were usually confined to, or directed into, separate activities from the mothers. There was a perceived need to provide male staff to engage effectively with male users. Both staff and users tended to define men's and women's needs as identifiably different, and sometimes in conflict.

For example, this manager said of her centre:

If we get a men's group going, it will be on a different day [when the women aren't here]. So then they can come down and use the same room that the mums use ... they'd do their own thing ... and we'll have a male facilitator. Then they can take ownership and that's their special time ... They [will get] the same esteem as the women get, the same time and space [but

Barriers to men's use of family centres

separately] *because the mothers are not keen for the dads to be down here on the same day.*

The agnostic approach
'Agnostic' centres had no identifiable approach. These centres appeared not to have formulated an explicit view about whether working with fathers required a particular approach or not.

Case example
Relatively few men were using these centres, except where they had been specifically referred. Activities were in principle open to all – like gender-blind centres the ethos was about everyone interacting together. Male users were, however, perceived as a rather unusual and unknown quantity. The issue of whether or how to accommodate male users was one which staff had either not really pursued in depth, or where there were ongoing, unresolved issues. There were no male staff. There was often a perception amongst staff and parents that men were inherently uninterested in greater involvement in parenting in general, and in accessing family centres in particular.

> For example, one worker said:
>
> *You can't just drag* [men] *in – they have got to want to come. Short of dragging them in, we can't do anything … The dads don't want to know.*
>
> *Q: Would it change the centre if more fathers started coming?*
>
> *I've never even thought of it, because we've never had men to worry about. We just plod on with whoever comes … and it's mainly just the mums.*

These three groupings cross-cut the five-fold typology outlined in Chapter 2. Additionally, some centres were divided into different and almost autonomous service components, so that traces of more than one orientation were discernible within the centre as a whole. Nevertheless, we found the groupings useful in understanding associations between individual centres and the experiences reported by respondents in respect of men's use of the centre.

We now describe in detail how family-centre-level barriers operated in three related areas of functioning:

- centre priorities and policies, including referral systems and staff and user attitudes to men

- the service provided, in terms of staffing and activities

- and, finally, the atmosphere and 'feel' of the centre.

Family centre priorities and policies
Family centre priorities and policies may impact on engagement with fathers and are reflected both in the way centres obtain users or clients and in the attitudes of staff and users to incoming men.

'It is more often the mother of a child that is referred' – referral policies and systems
The way family centres acquire their clientele (e.g. by referral or open-access) is an obvious factor in determining the extent to which fathers – at least in theory – have access to centres. Whilst 'open-access' centres should present no institutional barriers to the involvement of fathers, the referral systems common in 'child protection', 'day-care' and mixed-type centres could occasionally act as structural barriers. This was because referrals were often seen as

Fathers and family centres

applying to the mother and children only, thus effectively keeping fathers out.

> Q: *Why are there less fathers than mothers here?*
>
> I guess possibly because it is more often the mother of a child that is referred.
> (Female worker)
>
> Q: *Is there an issue about the project building a relationship with one person and seeing only that person as your client?*
>
> Yes I think so, and if it's [a] referred [case] and one person's referred in ... they don't refer [the partner].
>
> Q: *So the mother [gets] referred, not the father?*
>
> Yes. Because the health visitor will just work with the [mother], you know – [she'll say] *'I think there's an issue with the mother'*.
> (Female worker)

Of course, if access to a family centre is mediated by a more or less formal referral system, operated by external agencies, there may be relatively little the family centre itself can do to influence the number of fathers who are referred. However, we did find some evidence to suggest that centres with a 'gender-blind' and 'gender-differentiated' orientation (i.e. those which had a definite approach to working with men) tended to have more joint referrals than centres that were 'agnostic' in their approach to working with men. They also tended to regard use by women as a mandate to try to engage partners as well. On the other hand, centres with 'agnostic' tendencies (having no clear policy on working with men) were far more likely to be working with women alone. This suggests that having no clear approach is, of itself, a barrier to engaging with men.

'Sometimes the fathers cause stress with the mums' – attitudes and approaches to working with fathers

The extent to which fathers were seen as potential clients, or users, was also reflected in the attitudes of staff to working with men. As we discuss in the next chapter, the prevailing view across the sample as a whole was that it was generally desirable to engage fathers in family centre work. However, in talking about the specifics, rather than the generalities, of working with fathers, many staff cited areas of potential, or actual difficulty. Interestingly, where staff expressed particular reservations about working with men, existing users (and sometimes even non-users) often endorsed or echoed their views. What was not clear was who was influencing whom, though it seems likely that staff 'set the tone' for parents' attitudes to the work of the centre.

'We're dealing with domestic violence cases – the women need space from the men' – the risk of violence to women

The risk of violence was highlighted particularly in centres which catered to referred and especially disadvantaged families, where there was certainly a strong feeling that family centres were a 'safe haven' for vulnerable women. The feeling was that this could be damaged if men were allowed in.

In one 'gender-differentiated' centre, a worker explained why fathers had historically been excluded from some of sessions:

> My personal view was it wouldn't work [having men around] *because we're dealing with quite a few domestic violence cases. It really wasn't appropriate because the women need space from*

Barriers to men's use of family centres

the men and they would be unnerved by a man in the group.
(Female worker)

An uninvolved father from the same centre agreed, and felt strongly that he didn't have a place in the centre because of women's vulnerability:

I just don't think it's right that I should be involved 'cos ... if there's a woman that's got problems ... with men, from physical abuse and such from their partners or whatever, if a man goes down [to the family centre] *that woman's going to feel nervous, apprehensive, she's going to sit in the corner and not interact, and not take part ...*
(Steve, uninvolved father)

A mother who had herself been a victim of domestic violence expressed a similar view:

Obviously if the woman's been in a violent relationship she's very nervous of men. Frightened, even ... She wouldn't come here if there was a man here – she wouldn't do it ... I wouldn't have [in the past, though] *I would now, 'cos I'm over it, you know.* [But] *it takes a long time* [to get over it].
(Terri, mother, uninvolved partner)

Not surprisingly in a profession in which most staff are female, some workers were also concerned about the possible risks to staff of working with violent men:

We've had quite a few situations and it's been very intimidating for female members of staff to be faced with an angry man.
(Female worker)

Q: *Do you think it* [would] *make a difference to the kind of atmosphere of the place generally, having more men around?*

Make it more tense.

Q: *Tense for* [whom]?

[Laughter] *Everyone, I think. I mean I don't think it's an easy option, working with the men. I think it can create a lot of problems. I mean we had one incident ... it caused a lot of problems ...* [one man] *had a very, very violent history... And it all ended badly when he decided to threaten to kill me and we had to get the police involved ... It was an awful incident and it was an awful few months.*
(Female worker)

However, the same worker felt it was important to retain a sense of perspective about these sorts of incidents which, although frightening, were not common:

That was one particular incident – [but] *the other two violent men we've dealt with have responded and they're doing really well ...*

Other staff (often from centres with a 'gender-blind' orientation) commented that the risks from violent women could be just as great as those from men:

Q: *Are there any ... issues about having men around in the centre, any problems that have ever cropped up, or difficulties of any sort?*

... No, I haven't actually experienced any really, I mean I can't even say like the violent side of it, because the violent ones, their partners, the mums, are always violent as well, 'cos they're kind of violent together. So if you're in a ... volatile situation ... they're both likely to be violent rather than just the one. So I can't boil it down to it being a problem about having a man in the building.
(Female worker)

Fathers and family centres

'There's this spectre of male abuse which hangs over so many things' – danger to children

Another potential problem connected with men's use of family centres was related to a concern about children's safety. Not surprisingly, in centres where referred fathers had been accused of offences against children, staff commented that caution was essential and that inevitably such men could be prevented from using the centre to its full extent:

I think we have to be careful, depending on the reasons why they're coming here … Some of the men we've had referred have been Schedule One offenders, so we'd have to be careful.

Q: So how do you deal with those kinds of situations?

[In previous cases] they tended to bring them in at times when there weren't many other people around, sort of work it that way.
[Female worker]

But even where there was no genuine reason to treat a father in this way, as one worker commented, increasing public and professional awareness about child sexual abuse has meant that men who are interested in spending time with children may be regarded as having suspicious motives. The worker saw this as a definite barrier to fathers' engagement with family centres, which operated at two levels: firstly, in discouraging men from showing 'too much' interest in child-related activities; and, secondly, in making women users hostile to men using the centre.

It's very clear … to me that one of the impediments for fathers' groups happening in family centres in this community is the fear that men have about being connected in some way with their children. And that makes life very difficult because it … forms part of an unspoken agenda in [this area] at the moment … And one or two people have spoken to me about, about the fears that they would have both as men, about being involved in fathers' group, but also … some women have spoken about their suspicions of men being involved and … wanting to be more connected … with children. There's this spectre of male abuse which hangs over so many things.
(Male worker)

'A room full of queers and bible-bashers' – the 'wrong' sort of men

Apart from these perceptions of dangerousness, amongst some respondents there was also a feeling that the men who used centres might be in some way 'different' to most other men. Sometimes perceptions of men using centres were actively pejorative – indicating that male use of centres was so unusual as to be seen as deviant. Men who saw male users in this light were unlikely to want to be involved with a family centre.

This man described how he had imagined a men's group to be before he got involved:

I knew [someone who] come to a group like this, and I thought they were a bunch of tossers. A room full of queers and bible-bashers. That's what I really expected. The problem is stereotypes. I know what men are thinking out there, the same as what I was thinking before I come to the group: 'They're all gay and they're all bible-bashers'.
(Roy, involved father)

In other cases, the view was not so much that male users of centres were deviant in a threatening sense, but that nevertheless they were 'different' from most men, with special

Barriers to men's use of family centres

requirements and special orientations to family life. For example, that they were likely to be lone fathers, or men who were, for other reasons, unusually involved in family life and child-care (for example, as main carers), or especially sensitive and in touch with their 'feminine side' (as we shall see in the next chapter, this perception had some basis in fact):

Q: Would it ... take a certain type of bloke to go up there [to the family centre]?

Yeah, one that's wrapped round his wife's finger, told to get up there, or he's bored and lonely, hasn't got a job or something like that. That's the type of bloke that goes up. That's my own opinion.
(Darren, uninvolved father)

Q: Do you know any other blokes whose partners take their kids up there?

No ... If you're a feminine type of bloke and you gets on with women ... don't mind sit[ting] down and talk[ing] your head off with them, then you'd be all right – but I can't do that.
(Raymond, uninvolved father)

It looks like a particular man which comes [to the drop-in], you know. It's the men ... who you would see carrying their baby in like one of those ... baby sling things on their back or their front ... Yeah, I would think it was one of those sort of men ... They don't mind being seen doing it, and, you know, maybe changing the baby's nappy and that – they don't see it as a problem.
(Male worker)

'I wouldn't feel comfortable ...' – inhibiting effects on women users

Some interviewees felt that the presence of men in a family centre could make women feel uncomfortable or inhibited. This comment was typical of many workers' views:

I think you'll find that ... women wouldn't talk about things they might well talk about, if the men were there.
(Female worker)

Some mothers endorsed this perception, and linked it to what they saw as a male tendency to be patronising and disrespectful to women. In this centre – a strongly gender-differentiated one – men were allowed to visit, but were not allowed to participate in some of the weekday, women-only sessions. There were ongoing plans to start up some activities for fathers, but to take place on different days:

Q: What do you think would happen if the men ... were coming in [to the family centre] on the same day [as the women]?

I think it would be a bit funny.

Q: In what way?

They might take the mickey out of us ... Some blokes do.

Q: What sort of things might they say ...?

That you shouldn't do that or you shouldn't do this ... My partner does that.
(Angie, mother, involved partner)

One father agreed:

Sometimes the [men] causes stress with the mums ... they should change their attitude. One of the blokes [who comes here] talks to you like shit.
(Steve, uninvolved father)

In this 'agnostic' centre women were not used to having men around and, on the whole, didn't think this was such a bad thing:

17

Fathers and family centres

I don't think I could stay ... if there was loads of men there ... I wouldn't feel right. It feels relaxed and comfortable when we're up there. But if men were staying there, [if] the men was trying to have a chat with you, I think I'd [leave]. I don't know why. I wouldn't feel comfortable.
(Natalie, mother, uninvolved partner)

There were also issues of culture for some centres and for those working with women from Muslim backgrounds, the advantages of preserving 'women only' space in family centres was very much at the forefront of their concerns:

Q: What's the reaction of the women to having a man in the group, or men around?

Some people are very quiet. Especially [when] we had some women from Iraq and Iran ...It's their culture ... you don't speak [in front of men] ... You follow that system. So it stopped them opening up ... Women have a greater need [to use the centre] because women don't have anywhere else to go. Especially, I'm talking about the Bengali women here.
(Female worker)

'Mister Romeo at the playgroup' – sexual tensions and couple issues

The potential for sexual tensions, difficulties or embarrassments arising from men and women interacting with one another is rarely acknowledged in studies about working with men in a family support environment. However, we found that both staff and parents identified a number of potential problems of this sort, ranging in significance from minor irritations to more serious disincentives to men's involvement in family centres. For example, both staff and parents talked about the problem of flirting between male and female users – sometimes in relation to actual flirting and sometimes in relation to worries about being *accused* of flirting or 'taken the wrong way'.

This worker highlighted some of the problems of working with couples in a mixed sex environment:

Well there are some issues because you'll get a mum who will always think 'Phew, he's a bit of alright' and flashes her eyelashes, and then you've got the mother who's feeling a bit poorly and vulnerable, and this is an ongoing issue with a couple of our families at the moment. A mum's feeling at a low ebb, [and will] turn to a bottle because she's feeling pushed out ... so it has its disadvantages.
(Female worker)

And some fathers, both involved and uninvolved with family centre activities, talked about the 'flirting problem' and its effects:

You know I don't think [you see] many men in a place like this, [because] ... they would more or less think to themselves they [would] get a reputation 'Oh my God I can't go in there, it's all women – what are people going to say?' – you know, [that you're] a flirt or something ... 'there's mister Romeo ... he goes to the playgroup' ... I think it's one of the main [problems], to be quite honest with you.
(Dan, involved father)

One father (described as 'outgoing' by staff) in fact felt very inhibited by the fear of being 'taken the wrong way' by women users of the centre – so much so that he tended not to interact with them when he visited:

It's difficult to approach women, it's difficult to start up a conversation, because ... it's loaded,

Barriers to men's use of family centres

very often you don't really know how you're going to be taken and so generally what happens is, I've been coming here and keeping myself to myself for some time.
(Lloyd, involved father)

A usually uninvolved father who had taken part in a trip that the family centre had organised had got in trouble with his partner for talking to other women:

I don't feel at ease talking to women, 'cos like, the missus starts getting jealous and I get in trouble. Like when I went on that trip, she was asking me questions about who I was talking to … That does cause a lot of problems.
(Matthew, uninvolved father)

This mother felt some women would not want men around in the centre because of the sexual dimension that would be introduced to the atmosphere:

I don't mind [personally], but there's a lot of women [at the family centre] that would say 'No, we don't want men up here' …

Q: Why's that?

Because women are all right in an atmosphere with other women but [they] can feel self-conscious in front of men … So if there was more men up here they're going to think 'Oh I need to get all my nice clothes on, I need to do my hair, I need to do my make up', which isn't functional when you've got kids about anyway. [And] a lot of women can be jealous … 'She's looking at my man.' 'Cos obviously then that would cause a lot of arguments as well I think.
(Terri, mother, uninvolved partner)

In general, 'problematised' attitudes, such as those discussed above, tended to be most pronounced in the 'agnostic' centres, where both staff and parents talked rather dispiritedly about the problems of engaging with men. They tended to present these as more or less insoluble, rooted in the broader society, in local cultures and in 'men's natures'. For example, in agnostic centres parents made these comments:

I don't think there's much you can change about it because the men just wouldn't come anyway. I just don't think they can be bothered with the family centre.
(Sheena, mother, involved partner)

I don't think there's a great deal they can do to pull the men in … It's a very much male dominant area … for men to … actually be involved … would be a big leap in the dark for them.
(Gavin, involved father)

On the other hand, centres with a gender-differentiated approach were also quite aware of the difficulties arising out of trying to work with men, although they tended to take a more problem-solving approach, often highlighting ways in which these barriers could be worked at or circumvented. Centres which took a 'gender-blind' approach were more likely to minimise the problems, or regard them as relatively unimportant.

Family centre services: staffing and activities

The service that is provided at a family centre, in terms of staffing (i.e. whether mixed, or women-only team) and activities on offer may also present barriers to the engagement of fathers. The lack of male staff was noticeable across the sample of centres as a whole, with only five centres having any male staff presence at all (including sessional workers) and none having more than one man on the staff team. Similarly, few centres in our sample were seen as having a great deal to offer to fathers in terms of activities.

'There's nobody to relate to on the men's side' – the absence of male workers

The issue of whether lack of male staff actually creates a barrier to men's engagement with family centres is currently a topic of heated debate amongst practitioners and a subject which probably merits a study in its own right. Our findings in this respect were mixed, though many people thought the absence of male workers was generally regrettable.

> I think if they had more male teachers [i.e. staff] as well, I think that would bring more fathers in, 'cos they'd have someone to relate to. At the minute it's just [there's] nobody to relate to on the men side, sort of thing. It's just a bit strange.
> (Matthew, uninvolved father)

> I think there should be more male workers actually, but you don't see many that's working here. But I think if a fella's talking to a fella about their problem, then I think they'll open up more than what they would to a female. Yeah, I think there should be more male workers working in the system.
> (Shelley, mother, uninvolved partner)

'There's nothing for us up there, is there?' – the service(s) and activities provided by family centres

In fact, irrespective of the presence of male staff, the lack of activities catering to men was frequently mentioned by all groups of respondents – men, women and staff – and seemed to be a highly significant barrier to men becoming regular users of family centres. The majority of both men and women who took part in the study were convinced that, until family centres provided activities more suitable for or acceptable to men, few fathers would be seen on the premises on a regular basis.

It was sometimes difficult to disentangle respondents' feelings about the *service* provided by centres and their views of the more general *character* of the place. This was a particular problem because of the overwhelming sense of feminisation, common to all centres, which coloured perceptions of all aspects of a centre's functioning. This is discussed in more detail in the next section. Yet, perhaps one of the most interesting findings to arise out of the study was an important distinction between the provision of *activities* (in terms of the specific 'things to do' that were on offer) and the provision of *activity* in a generic sense. In terms of *activities*, men found many of the organised activities on offer at family centres highly gendered and of little interest. Furthermore, a major shortcoming of family centres was described as the lack of *activity* on offer, in terms of opportunities to engage in activity which was seen as physical (i.e. 'active' as opposed to 'passive'), constructive and meaningful to men.

'It's just not my scene' – attitudes to gendered activities

The organised *activities* offered by centres, many of which were reported to be greatly enjoyed by women (for example, sewing, making Christmas decorations, glass painting, aromatherapy) were not, on the whole, of much interest to fathers. Though many staff claimed that men did enjoy these traditionally 'women's' activities, we found few fathers willing to confirm this:

Barriers to men's use of family centres

There's nothing here for men. It's like they do courses on aromatherapy, and things – it's not the type of thing you want to do, you know.

Q: There are some blokes who do aromatherapy though aren't there?

I'm sure there are! I just wouldn't like to do it myself. Just not my scene you know.
(Rod, uninvolved father)

It's not my thing, you know? ... I mean ... sort of making Christmas decorations and things like that ... it's not the sort of thing a man's going to [do] ... well, it's weird!
(Joe, uninvolved father)

Although in some centres staff insisted that past experience confirmed that men could be induced to participate in and enjoy 'women's' activities, others felt this was something of a misapprehension:

It's seen as ... politically correct: that if females can have their nails and hair done, there's no reason why the men can't have theirs done. But in reality, men don't want their nails or their hair doing. I don't think the men see it [in the same way] as ... maybe the management [do] ... I don't think men see it as being OK ... I think sometimes it's probably our own little fantasy world ...

Q: Have any of the men made comments to you about the ... activities?

Yeah they have, 'oh that's not for me' sort of thing, and [when those activities are about to start] that's when they [leave] ... 'Oh God', they probably have said, ' I'm not staying for this.' Even though they are invited [to stay].
(Male worker)

It was also suggested that the lack of anything to do apart from playing with children was found boring by a lot of men:

I don't know what my partner would like to do really ... I know he finds it a bit boring because ... you only play with the child and stuff. I think he'd like to do something different – he does get bored.
(Diane, mother, involved partner)

'He's more of a hands-on person' – activities with a practical application

Men also wanted activities that were useful, skills-based and had a wider practical application, as the examples below show.

Q: What would you like to see them doing here?

Showing people how to use computers – that'd be perfect, that'd be brilliant. How to use the Internet, for example, you know important things, things that are going to [affect] everyday life ... Art as well ... Language skills, communications. I'd even see if I could get someone in to teach people a foreign language. Give 'em a bit of self-esteem. Something that they wouldn't normally do, or wouldn't normally dream of. Something to whet the appetite, so that then they could think 'mmmm, I'm good at this, I'd like to do more' – and then I'd pursue a college course.
(Steve, uninvolved father)

I think Dave would probably come if there was something ... for him to do, you know rather than just sit around having a brew ... He's more of a hands-on person ... If he could make a coffee table or a whatever, I think he would tend to want to come more then.
(Kirsty, mother, uninvolved partner)

Fathers and family centres

As we show in the next chapter, where there were insufficient opportunities for this kind of constructive activity, men were sometimes described as creating them, as if in an attempt to give themselves a 'role' where one did not exist. This may reflect stereotypical expectations of men and men's roles in a family environment; however, the sheer number of times this issue was spontaneously mentioned by men, women and centre staff convinced us that lack of this kind of practical activity needs to be taken seriously, as a barrier to greater male interest in family centres.

'Talking about nothing, wasting the day away' – the lack of constructive activity

In terms of *activity*, sitting around, drinking coffee, watching children play and talking with other parents (something women in family centres spend a lot of time engaged in) was not, on the whole, something men enjoyed or saw the value of. They found it frustratingly passive, characterised it as 'gossiping' and saw it as essentially pointless and unconstructive:

Sitting down, talking about nothing, wasting the day away: I got better things to do in the day.

Q: That's what happens is it, at the family centre, they just talk about nothing?

They just talk about ... anything and everything. Women's talk ... If they want to talk about things like that I'll just go home and do things. I say ... to myself 'Why am I here talking a load of rubbish when I could be at home working, do something, cleaning up the house?'... I'm always working, I can't just sit down and talk, talk and talk, drink coffee, talk and talk ... they seems to go and sit there and drink tea and smoke fags and talk their heads off. I ain't up for that.
(Dan, involved father)

Me, my topic of conversation is cars – men things. I can't see them [women] wanting to talk about that kind of thing. It's just ... gossip and women gossip[ing] amongst each other [at the family centre]. I've got nothing to gossip about.
(Matthew, uninvolved father)

And though men agreed that 'just talking' was what men typically did in the pub, they added that the subjects of conversation there were different to those thought suitable within a family centre!

Q: But blokes ... chat together up the pub?

Ah that's [different], we talk about sport and sex, or women.
(Darren, uninvolved father)

'They want manly sports, like football' – the lack of physical activity

What many men bemoaned above all was a lack of activity at family centres in the physical sense of the word – for example, active games like football, and things they could do with children and with other men that involved physical exertion. Being indoors all the time was also described as frustrating by some men.

Q: And did your partner go down to the drop-in as well or was that something you just did yourself?

No, I think he likes the baby gym at [town] more, because that was more of an active thing. And the drop-in at [the family centre] was just like sitting on a chair, and was really, really boring [for him] ... It's just not geared for men, really.
(Diane, mother, involved partner)

Q: What would get more men to come here?

I'd say ... get them to come in to five-a-side football, because then they would start coming ... so that when you come back you can sit down,

Barriers to men's use of family centres

have a good team chat about the game ... you can get the men in but you've got to look at it totally different than what they [the family centre] are doing. They're looking at it from a woman's point of view, what a woman wants to do, aerobics and things like that. Blokes don't want that. They want manly sports like football, five-a-side and stuff like that ... So, you've got to say well, look from a man's [point of view], what does a man want in here?
(Phil, involved father)

'It's not my thing, men chatting together' – dedicated men's activities

It is sometimes assumed that the provision of a 'men's group' (in the sense of a men-only discussion group) is the panacea that will remedy the absence of men in centres, and that, once men's groups are provided, fathers will feel catered for, welcomed and generally more engaged with family centres. In the next chapter, we discuss how dedicated men's activities can indeed be regarded by some men as incentives to use family centres.

But, as our team quickly found, men's groups do not appeal to all men. The few men's groups that we came across tended to be poorly or sporadically attended (with one exception) and several had petered out over the course of time. None seemed be integrated more than superficially with the other elements of the centre, with all operating more or less autonomously. This meant that men attending the groups might not have any contact with other services provided by the centre, or even seem very aware of what else the centre did. Conversely, involved men using other parts of these services (e.g. referred fathers doing 'programme' work, or using an open-access drop-in) and uninvolved partners of women using the centres often claimed to be completely unaware that a men's group actually existed within the centre. Whilst we recognise that this may not be typical of all men's groups and that well-known examples of 'good practice' and highly successful groups exist within some family centres, our study suggested that it is a mistake to see provision for fathers as beginning and ending with men's groups.

From the outside, many men expressed doubts that men's groups would work, and seemed unlikely to be persuaded to try one:

Q: How do you feel about the idea of a [men's] discussion group ...? What sort of picture comes to mind?

I don't know what to think. I don't see what they actually get to talk about. I can't see there being a topic of conversation. I think it'd just be like they'd all go in and ... just talk about – just owt really. I can't see [them] talking about kids ...
(Matthew, uninvolved father)

I'd say it's not my thing. Men chatting together. What I told my wife, I don't want to hear bloody blokes talking, and most of them [other men] will tell you the same.
(Darren, uninvolved father)

Q: What do you think it would be like just ... talking, just with a bunch of men, but not in a pub?

Very strange, yeah, very strange. The sports activities and clubs is what we've always done like me and my mates, it's always been that and ... instead of a cup of tea, a pint. You just go into a room, just to have a chat? That seems strange to me.
(Neil, uninvolved father)

Fathers and family centres

In summary, the absence of both male staff and activities appealing to men was extremely widespread. This made it difficult to assess the extent to which this created a barrier to engaging fathers in centres with different orientations. However, centres with an 'agnostic' orientation were probably regarded as the least appealing to men on this count. This was not surprising perhaps; these tended to be the centres with no male staff and where the issue of whether fathers would find the activities provided in the centre attractive had rarely even been considered. However, gender-blind centres were also described as failing men in this regard. Perhaps because of the explicit ethos of 'non-differentiation' in these centres, male staff (where they existed) were not encouraged to relate to male users in a gender-specific way, thus perhaps missing an opportunity to establish stronger bonds with male users. The activities in these centres, whilst often described by staff as gender-neutral, were often not perceived as such by users and tended secretly to be regarded with disdain by many fathers. On the other hand, gender-differentiated centres were the most likely to try and provide services and staff specifically for fathers, and in some respects were least likely to be criticised for failing to cater to men. However, the equation of 'men's activities = men's groups', which often pertained in these centres, meant that fathers who were not interested in discussion groups were also not catered for.

Family centre atmosphere and 'feel'
We have discussed the barriers presented by different aspects of family centre structure, and what is provided by centres in terms of activities and staffing. However, the 'feel' of a family centre – the way it was perceived by men and the general 'atmosphere' of the place – turned out to be perhaps the most significant barrier of all in preventing men from attending centres on a regular basis. Even amongst those men who were already attending centres fairly regularly, many spoke of the 'feel' of the centre, as something which almost certainly discouraged other men from getting more fully involved in the centre's activities.

Most important of all, every centre in the sample was described by respondents as feeling significantly 'feminised' – that is, as being women-dominated and as a place whose primary function was to cater to women (or women and children). This single factor was probably the most frequently mentioned issue for fathers and virtually all other barriers described as arising out of the feel, or atmosphere, of a centre flowed from this.

'They might as well just call it the "female centre" ' – feminised environment
Given the preponderance of women in family centres, both as users and as staff, it will not surprise anyone that our study confirmed the picture reported elsewhere of family centres as 'women's places' (e.g. Smith, 1996). Almost by definition, the fact that women dominate numerically (as in most family support contexts) would be expected to lead to a general perception of 'feminisation'. The mere fact that men were so outnumbered in most centres that we visited led, for some, to a perception that the purpose of the centre must be to cater for mothers. Some men felt that this was right and proper – that mothers' needs were greater than fathers' and that, by implication, fathers had a

Barriers to men's use of family centres

lesser claim to the use of the centre. It seems plausible to expect that these perceptions would act as substantial discouragements to men using family centres:

> *I think the centre [is] for children, mothers and fathers. But, in practice, what I see is there's many, many more women here, so I don't know, maybe it is intended for women – mothers and babies.*
> (Lloyd, involved father)

> *The male way of thinking is, if you walk into an environment that's all women, that's all that should be there.*
> (Neil, uninvolved father)

> *They may as well just [call it] the 'female centre'. It must be quite intimidating for men coming in here with all these women. I wouldn't like it if I was a female and there was loads of men.*
> (Female worker)

Some respondents thought that the reactions of staff to men's rare appearances at family centres compounded this sense of being slightly unwelcome:

> *I think the staff have a bit of difficulty dealing with ... fathers who come in here. I don't think they mean to do that ... they're just not used to fathers coming in there ... What I find is they don't welcome him as much as they would a mother who came into the place ... When a mother comes in they would ... give her a good introduction and walk around the place and show them exactly what we do, and I don't see the males getting that ... So ... I think ... the female workers ... feel a bit apprehensive when a male comes in.*
> (Male worker)

Some days it's 'slagging off men day' here – hostility to men

We were struck by the far-reaching implications and often surprisingly concrete and tangible effects of this feminisation, not only in terms of how centres were perceived in a general sense but also in how they were experienced on a day-to-day basis by the men and women we interviewed. For example, in some centres, both men and women described the behaviour of women users towards men as being actively problematic. Women were described as unfriendly, unwelcoming, or even overtly hostile towards men, as if they felt the presence of a male somehow undermined the cosy atmosphere of the centre. Not surprisingly, this was described as discouraging fathers from making full use of the centre.

Recounting his occasional forays into the drop-in provided by his local family centre, this father said:

> *I get the impression that I'm a man and I shouldn't be there. I should be a mother with my toddler and I'd be welcome ...*
> (Roy, involved father)

> *It's probably difficult for men to go down there, especially with all the other women 'cos [it's] as though you're like a social outcast ...'What's he doing here?'*
> (Simon, uninvolved father)

Women and staff also endorsed these perceptions:

> *When he [partner] used to come in with me, they'd talk to me but they wouldn't talk to him. So he felt like he was ostracised and he felt, and I picked up on it as well, that it was almost a hostile environment – that he was dismissed*

Fathers and family centres

because he was the father and I was the mother.
(Judy, mother, involved partner)

You can come in here and basically it's 'slagging off men day'.
Q: What, among the staff, or among the service users?
Everyone.
(Female worker)

'He'd just go red …' – sexual harassment of male users

As we described earlier, both staff and parents commented on occasional sexual tensions which were seen as an inevitable by-product of having both women and men using family centres. In some cases, the risk of being accused of having ulterior, sexual motives for using a family centre was perceived as a definite barrier to men's greater involvement in centre activities. However, some comments suggested that, rather than being seen as predatory, the greatest risk run by a father using some of the centres in the sample was the reverse situation: falling victim to what can only be described as sexual harassment by women users. In most cases this was described as more in the nature of 'flirting' and a minor irritation or embarrassment for the men. Indeed, many men seemed at pains to insist that they could 'cope' with this sort of behaviour. However, in other cases the behaviour was described as intimidating and highly off-putting to male users:

We had, last year, a couple of excursions with the kids … and they enjoyed it tremendously.
Q: And what did you get out of it?
Oh [laughter], what did I get? I got a couple of women who had a crush on me … and I felt embarrassed.
Q: So there was … flirting going on, was there?
Yes, it was and I felt embarrassed … I think it was a compliment but I felt embarrassed because [people] were listening … and I felt uneasy …
(Victor, involved father)

When Paul was here we used to rag him … talk about sex in front of him … poor old Paul is sitting there, listening to all this, reading his paper … If it was the other way round it could be [called] sexual harassment.
(Female worker)

Again, we had a single male [using the session]. And what we had was flirting, and the poor guy … he was very shy and [the mothers] would just embarrass him most of the time [laughter].
Q: Would they tease him or …?
Yeah, teasing him, we had some that were very outspoken and quite crude …
Q: Did they make … sexual jokes and innuendo and things?
Yeah, yeah.
Q: And how did that affect him do you think?
Well he just used to go red …
(Female worker)

A man that is here [using the family centre] now … he does get embarrassed at the things the women talk about. He's getting used to us now but he used to get very embarrassed … [there was a] woman that was breast feeding [who] was not tactful at all … she … offered to let him drink some milk if he wanted it. It was on his first day up here as well, I felt very sorry for him. I honestly did not think he'd come back again.
(Terri, mother, uninvolved partner)

Barriers to men's use of family centres

***'They're a bit like dinosaurs at the moment, the fathers – a rare breed'* – the absence of other male users**

If the physical predominance of women in family centres created some barriers to involving fathers more fully then, conversely, the physical absence of men was also perceived as a barrier in its own right. Even when non-users of centres could think of little else to account for their lack of involvement or interest in family centres, the conspicuous absence of other males was frequently cited as a major issue.

That's the one downfall of that place that there is not enough blokes, it's like all women. Puts you on edge.
(Matthew, uninvolved father)

It'd be nice to me if there was other fathers going to this thing, and I'd go along with them … I feel sort of on the spot, when there's so many mothers and things like that.
(Joe, uninvolved father)

They're a bit like dinosaurs at the moment, the fathers. I mean it's a rare breed.
(Male worker)

Even regular family centre users could feel intimidated by the lack of any other male presence:

I think there was only one other dad went on the trip. It was all women, and I was more or less the only father that was there.

Q: How does that make you feel when you're the only father there?

A bit uncomfortable really because you're sat there on the coach and all you hear is all these women gaggling around you and the kids screaming and bawling, and you think to yourself 'what the heck am I doing here'?
(Derek, involved father)

A by-product of rarity value, when a man made an appearance, he was often described as being subject to overt scrutiny by women. Though essentially benign, the slightly critical flavour of this scrutiny cannot have added to the fathers' sense of comfort.

But it's such a shock when you see a man come into the room. That's unusual, it's like an alien or something! … I think [men] feel really uncomfortable, but it's only because it's unusual – that's the only thing really.

Q: What is it, do you think, that makes the men feel a bit uncomfortable?

When you come here everybody watches each other … you look [at] the way people are doing things with their child, definitely, and it's very competitive. I think, personally I tend to look at what fathers do more, maybe. Because it's unusual to see men doing that … so you are watching more I think. Well I am.

Q: What for exactly?

Well, the way they do things, say like giving their child a drink … if they do it in the right order as I'd do it, say, or if they do it differently because they're not used to it. And also [for] being there if they need a hand as well, if their child was screaming.
(Diane, mother, involved partner)

***'You watch your Ps and Qs when there's a woman sitting there'* – not being able to relax**

Finally and perhaps not surprisingly, given the extent to which men in family centres appeared to be under scrutiny, another 'atmospheric'

Fathers and family centres

barrier that we uncovered related to fathers' sense of 'not being able to be yourself' as a man in a family centre. For some men, as we have seen, the tensions were sexual in nature; but, for others, the problems arose out of perceptions of the different public behaviours of men and women. Some men felt that the centre was an unrelaxing environment, in which you had to be on your best behaviour. Bad language and certain 'male' topics of conversation (women and football were mentioned) were felt to be inappropriate, making some fathers feel ill at ease and tongue-tied. The presence of so many women 'in charge' and so many small children at the family centre reminded some men of school (another place where you have to behave yourself!) – even to the extent of calling the day-care staff 'teachers'.

(In a mixed group) …The men have got a different way of talking together. When you are with a woman you have to … think of what you're saying sometimes.
(Victor, involved father)

I mean it's like school up there, in a way, isn't it?
Q: What is it that gives you that impression?
Because … it's not the sort of place you go to discuss sex, or women, or football … 'Cos it's run by women, one. Two, they haven't got a bar up there. And, three, you couldn't swear. It's like a school, all women running it … talking quiet.
(Darren, uninvolved father)

This man described how the men's group he attended changed when a woman worker came in:

Q: How's it different when she's here?
I don't swear as much …You know, you sort of watch your Ps and Qs when there's a … woman sitting there.
(Darren, uninvolved father)

As we have shown, the effects of feminisation were widespread and far-reaching. The centres which were seen as most female-dominated and least man-friendly tended to be the 'agnostic' group of centres – but neither gender-blind nor gender-differentiated centres were immune from criticism. The self-reported experience of men in centres that claimed to have a 'gender-neutral' approach was often inconsistent with the centre's expressed aims, because men still felt excluded. Even in centres with dedicated men's activities and a specific recognition of fathers as having separate needs from those of mothers, the effects of feminisation were still felt to be very much in evidence in the main body of the centre.

4 Enabling factors in men's use of family centres

Introduction

In the previous chapter we identified a range of barriers which appeared both to prevent fathers from attending family centres in the first place, and which made them uncomfortable or ill-at-ease once inside. However, whilst it was certainly the case that in all the family centres in our study women users vastly outnumbered the men, we found that some men *do* go to family centres and *are* able to engage – to a greater or lesser extent – with the services provided. In fact, there was some male presence found in every centre in the sample, although the extent of men's involvement varied considerably from the solitary male picking up a child from playgroup, through fathers undergoing child protection assessment procedures, to a flourishing men's group. In this chapter we look at some of the factors which help to make it possible for those 'involved' fathers to actually attend and engage with centres.

Enabling factors proved harder to isolate than barriers. This is partly because it is often easier to say why one *doesn't* do something than why one does. But, partly, it reflects the fact that enabling factors are not necessarily the mirror image of barrier factors and the absence of a particular barrier does not automatically create an 'enabling' environment. Rather, enabling factors appeared to operate in a subtle and cumulative way, acting independently of, or in parallel to, barriers. Thus, for example, in trying to understand why one man had been 'enabled' whilst another had not, it often appeared that two or three enabling factors had interacted to outweigh the effect of one particularly significant barrier.

The social and cultural context

In the previous chapter we referred to the prevalence of 'traditional' social attitudes, held by both men and women, to male roles in relation to child-care and parenting. It was also suggested that men's attitudes to family support services may be especially negative. However, such views were not universally held. There can be no doubt that many 'traditional' attitudes are, at least for some, undergoing change.

For example, several fathers contrasted their approach to being a parent with that of their own, absent, or emotionally distant father, and some family centre workers were also able to identify differences in attitude and practice between fathers of different generations. In more practical terms, several fathers (and mothers) described taking a shared or equal approach to domestic chores and parenting within the home, regardless of the employment status of either parent.

Though some negative attitudes were held by men towards family support services, these were by no means universal. For some fathers, engagement with family centres was the only means by which they could work towards gaining access to, or indeed have any contact at all with, their children. Others referred to the role that the centres (or individual workers within them) had played in keeping their families together and were quite open in acknowledging that they had – at some point – needed outside help and support. This was particularly true of lone fathers.

Fathers and family centres

Individual circumstances and motivations

Whilst many men did indeed feel that family centres had little to offer them as individuals, lone fathers and fathers who were the main carer for their children were, by contrast, often actively seeking the kind of social and practical support traditionally offered by centres to mothers and their children. Compared with most men, such fathers were in unusual circumstances and were often quite socially isolated. Reminiscent of accounts of why many women use family centres (e.g. Pithouse and Holland, 1999), these men spoke of being bored, stressed, lonely and needing to get themselves and their children out of the house.

As with barrier factors, another enabling factor operating at the individual level appeared to be related to individual orientations and 'personality' characteristics. It certainly seemed that it was easier for certain sorts of men to be accepted and to feel comfortable within a family-centre setting than others. Having stereotypically 'feminine' qualities, such as gentleness, an interest in children, or the ability to interact comfortably with women – or at the very least a willingness to become 'one of the girls' – was felt to be helpful in gaining acceptance within the feminised environment of many family centres. As one man put it:

> [Coming here] *I'm the oddity ... there's not many men ... like I am.*
> (Gavin, involved father)

Whilst having something of a 'female' side is certainly an enabling factor, determination, a degree of persistence and a thick skin also appear to be required during the process of gaining acceptance and recognition within some particularly female-dominated centres:

> *Part of coming here is not being bothered by other people's attitudes really, you know.*
> (Lenny, involved father)

Enabling factors at the family centre level

Enabling factors operating at the societal or individual levels are clearly important in helping us understand how some fathers can, given the right circumstances, become encouraged to get involved with family centres. However, cultural, social and individual level factors did not, on their own, account for the differences we found between centres, in terms of their record of success in engaging fathers. Family-centre-level enabling factors, as with barriers, turned out to be far more significant.

We did not set out with the expectation of finding centres which had discovered the key to successfully engaging large numbers of fathers. However, we did find plenty of pockets of success, albeit sometimes limited in scope or depth, and occasionally brought about by accident rather than by design. As with barrier factors, we found relatively little association between the 'type' of centre and either the existence or absence of factors which 'enabled' fathers' involvement. However, the three broad 'orientations' towards work with men (gender-blind, gender-differentiated and agnostic) were again useful in accounting for at least some of the differences between centres. Again, we approached our analysis of enabling factors at three related levels: policies and priorities; the service provided; and the atmosphere within centres.

Family centre priorities and policies

Notwithstanding the range of difficulties

Enabling factors in men's use of family centres

encountered, or anticipated, by staff in their attempts to work with men, the general view of family centre workers was that working with men was – in principle – a good thing to do. However, centres varied in the degree to which they endorsed this principle and were at various stages of development in terms of actually putting principles into practice. Indeed, for some centres (mostly the centres with an agnostic approach) it was not a priority at all. They were happy to carry on as they were, allowing men to use the centre if they turned up, but not actively pursuing the involvement of more men. Others, however, were actively pursuing or developing this side of their work, the gender-differentiated centres being most notable for this.

'They're shoved into it by social services' – referral policies and systems

Although we were not able to explore this area in great depth, the referral policies and systems of different centres appeared to be significant in influencing (although not determining) the extent and nature of fathers' involvement. Open-access centres, with their non-stigmatising approach (Pugh, 1992), are often thought to be easier to access than closed, referral-based services. In fact, in the case of fathers, we found that 'referral only' centres or parts of centres were on the whole *more* likely to be working with men. For example, if a centre took referrals where the whole family was viewed as the 'client', then fathers, where present in the family, would inevitably be found within that centre. At a basic level, treating referrals as family-based, rather than mother-and-child-based, can be regarded as an enabling factor; not only does it bring fathers through the door of the centre, but ensures that they participate in the activities therein.

> [The centre's] *always been available to work with men, but it's just that there's not been very many men available. But the nature of the work is changing and we are really getting involved with a lot of court assessment work* [now]. *If dads are on the scene they become part of that. So I think the reason we're working more with dads is because they're probably shoved into it by social services.*
> (Female worker)

However, there was some doubt as to whether some referred fathers got 'engaged' with the centre in more than a superficial way:

> Q: *Do you feel you have to go? What would happen if you just said 'I'm not going anymore'?*
>
> *Then it goes against us ... It goes back to social services and they would get annoyed, if we don't attend there, then the kids go in care.* [I] *would stop going if we didn't have to.*
> (Trevor, involved father)

We found that many referred men tended to stick closely to the terms of their programme of work or assessment, and tended not to become involved with other activities (such as courses or drop-in facilities) if any were available at the centre. This is a partly a further reflection of the general difficulty and discomfort experienced by fathers in joining in with open-access services, as discussed in some detail in Chapter 3, although similar 'ghettoisation' of referred families in mixed-type family centres has been commented on elsewhere (Smith, 1996).

Fathers and family centres

'The management has a lot to do with it' – setting priorities at management level

Explicit support at a managerial or centre policy level for the inclusion of fathers in the centre was mentioned by some staff and users as an important enabling factor, in terms of giving an impetus to new developments and in demonstrating a strong inclusive ethos. Inevitably, agnostic centres were not featured amongst the centres demonstrating strong support at management level to working with fathers. However, some centres with gender-blind or gender-differentiated orientations displayed evidence of commitment at policy or managerial level to these kinds of developments.

In this emphatically gender-blind centre, clear leadership from the manager ensured that staff were well aware of policies and priorities for working with all clients, including men.

> I think the management has a lot to do with it. We're lucky [manager's] really 'equal everything': She's [into] children's rights, we do consumer rights, we do anti-discriminatory practice all the time ... I think we're quite a lucky centre.
> (Female worker)

Men's groups, located within gender-differentiated centres, could only be successfully established with the backing of management. In one centre, the managerial commitment to working with fathers was demonstrated symbolically, by the physical allocation of space within the centre.

> At the outset we had a manager of the family centre here who was very, very keen for fathers ... to be involved in the life of the family centre and part of that involvement was that she would like to have had a fathers' group. And that was her agenda, she was very clear about that. And she put the fathers' group slap bang in the centre, quite symbolically, because we use the central room here.
> (Male worker)

In this centre, management support was provided by encouraging all staff to 'internally refer' fathers to the men's group.

> The way that we get men [to the group] is either they come to this drop-in here or they come with a partner and they're encouraged to get involved by the family centre staff, because they see it as a priority. We've had a lot of support from [management] and all the other staff ... so we rely on them to talk to the fathers.
> (Male worker)

'We've got to be objective ...and encourage them' – staff attitudes to working with men

As the quote above illustrates, positive managerial aspirations have also to be translated on the ground into positive staff attitudes to involving men if they are to be truly enabling. A commitment to this approach was visible in this statutory-run centre with a gender-blind orientation, as observed by one of the mothers:

> Here, they're really big on dad playing the part, and that's one thing. They really look at the family, not 'mum's done this' or 'dad's done that'.
> (Kelly, mother)

> The men have got to feel valued, it doesn't matter what we think about them, they've got to feel that they're the fathers of these children, whether we think they're capable or not of being good fathers. We've got to be very objective with them, and encourage them. They need valuing as much as the women do.
> (Female worker)

Enabling factors in men's use of family centres

'Pestering me to come down' – being proactive about getting men involved

A positive staff attitude to working with men is, on its own, relatively weak as an enabling factor. We found a number of centres where the staff said very positive things about working with men that did not seem to have impacted upon the users. Again, good intentions need to be translated into action.

Where centres had managed to involve fathers in any numbers, or had succeeded in engaging with them at anything more than a superficial level, there was generally evidence of some specific, focused action on the part of workers that had enabled this to come about. We found that one of the most effective means of getting men into and involved with family centres was through a personal introduction. This required willingness on the part of staff to build a relationship with the father on his own terms and often, initially, away from the family centre itself.

> *I don't think that we've worked with any families where the father hasn't engaged with us in some way ... But he might not necessarily attend* [the centre]. *I had one where I went out* [to him]. *We identified that father needed to be part of the work, so I went out after work, when he got home from work, and I'd go into the home and do it.*
> (Female worker)

It also required persistence and, of course, management support and resources. This involved father was now a regular attender at a men's group, but had to be asked 'hundreds' of times before he had joined in:

> *They asked me hundreds upon hundreds of times 'Do you fancy coming down?'* [and I'd say] *'No, no I'm not going to a place like that'.*
> (Roy, involved father)

However, there was some evidence to suggest extra effort might pay off. These uninvolved fathers thought a personal approach might just persuade them into their local centres:

> *I wouldn't turn them down if they asked me to go along.*
> (Joe, uninvolved father)

> *I think ... you are frightened to go in the first place ... you need that little push to go. I still believe that if people who'd run* [it] *came round and spoke to you and saw you then it'd probably encourage you to come down. I think that would help a lot.*
> (Simon, uninvolved father)

This uninvolved father, who had visited a centre once or twice and told us he was 'thinking' about getting further involved was, it seemed, definitely open to persuasion:

> *Q: You said this place was mainly for women and yet there are quite a few men who pop in now and again. What gets them to come in?*
>
> *Nosiness ... and the fact that Brenda does invite people ...* [I went] *because she is always asking me to be there; always ... pestering me to come down.*
>
> *Q: If she hadn't have 'phoned you would you still have come in?*
>
> *Probably not, I'd have probably just still stayed away.*
> (Steve, uninvolved father)

Staff who had tried this approach stressed the level of persistence required:

Fathers and family centres

> *Oh yes, it's very difficult, I mean when we first started there was a large turnover and sometimes there would be no men turn up to the meetings, sometimes one. I had to show persistence and commitment and I had to gain the trust of the men that, no matter what, I'll be there on that [day]. If they don't turn up I'll still be there.*
> (Male worker)

The above examples illustrate the challenge of getting fathers involved with family centres at 'entry-level'. However, continued effort is required to ensure a deeper level of engagement. This father was initially a most reluctant referral to a centre, but responded to the efforts of a worker to engage him:

> *At first I felt 'I don't want to be here ... end of story' ... [but] the project leader that was here put her faith in [me] ... and it was basically because somebody gave me a chance to put things right and had faith in me ... and, as I say, now I live here!*
> (Jack, involved father)

Approaching and encouraging fathers' involvement via their partners was – occasionally – successful.

> *As regards the family centre, it was Judy [partner] ... that sort of pushed me to go there, because ... me going into a female environment, that is ... a strange thing to do.*
> (Graham, involved father)

Where women expressed a desire that their partners become involved with the family centre, staff sometimes encouraged them to try and persuade their partners to visit – a sort of 'pyramid selling'. Such an approach could act as a definite enabling factor, at least in as far as getting the man through the door of the centre, even if no further. However this strategy could backfire if fathers' expectations were not met:

> *There used to be men going up there [to the family centre], and I said to [partner], 'Why don't you come up if there's others going up?', [but] when he did he was the only man there. So he said I conned him, [and] he wouldn't go again.*
> (Lisa, mother, uninvolved partner)

One worker describes a successful strategy by which a flourishing mixed group was developed. In this case, pyramid selling by partners used the promise of other men's presence as 'bait' to attract more fathers.

> *This group I'm talking about – I'd had this one family that I'd already been working with, and he [the father] came because he knew me and he'd worked with me ... And on the back of him coming, various girls who'd got partners at home would say [to them] 'Well, Mike goes, so why don't you come along?' And [the men] knew there was going to be another bloke there, and that's what brought them along.*
> (Female worker)

In terms of our orientation groupings, in agnostic centres we found little evidence of positive staff or management attitudes, or proactive behaviour which encouraged fathers' participation, despite a general agreement that, in principle, fathers ought to be more engaged with the centre. Indeed, all the examples discussed above are taken from centres which had taken some sort of definite 'stance', in terms of the way in which they were aiming to include men in the centre. Having such a commitment (irrespective of whether this was premised on minimising or stressing the gender gap) enabled staff to work proactively in engaging men,

Enabling factors in men's use of family centres

where necessary supporting flexibility in working arrangements to facilitate this – for example, by making home visits, or finding ways to accommodate women and men in different parts of the centre.

Family centre services: staffing and activities

'There are some things you can't talk to a woman about' – male staff

In terms of the service offered by family centres, we discussed in Chapter 3 the extent to which the absence of male staff in family centres could act as a barrier to working with male users. This is an area of some debate, which would benefit from more attention than we were able to give it in this study. Our findings were that male staff clearly enabled some men to feel more comfortable and 'legitimate' within a centre. However, perhaps surprisingly, staff and mothers put more stress on the importance and value of having male workers around than did fathers.

Given that not all family centres are able, in the present climate, to secure male workers, it is worth stating that our evidence shows clearly that it is possible to involve fathers in family centres without having a male worker on board. We found several examples where this had occurred. Indeed many of the 'involved' fathers we interviewed had no experience of male staff in a family centre setting. Having managed to 'engage' with the centre without the benefit of a male member of staff, it was felt by several that the sex of the workers was irrelevant, so long as they were helpful and supportive.

Q: Do you think it's good to have both men and women staff in places like family centres, or does it not matter?

It doesn't matter. If you get a good personality member of staff then it's OK.
(Trevor, involved father)

Some fathers actively favoured women staff as 'good listeners':

Q: Do you find it just as easy to talk to a woman as to a man?

I think ... talking to a woman is more better than talking to a man, because women listen more than men do.
(Trevor, involved father)

Nevertheless, having men on the staff was generally thought to be positive, particularly in providing a point of reference for men entering a largely female environment. This male worker felt it important to take an active role in welcoming and supporting fathers who used the drop-in facility.

I ... welcome him. As I would do a female, basically, so no different. But I do tell him that, 'Not a lot of males come here and I hope that you're not going to be put off by that ... Any problems you get, come and see me.'

Q: Right, so you make yourself available for them?

Yeah. I think they need that sort of support in here when they come down, just to be told where everything is and what have you ... I think they need more support than the females there, being a minority group in the centre. Most definitely.
(Male worker)

Having a male staff presence can be used not only as an effective 'entry-level' enabler, in assisting a father across the threshold, but also to engage fathers at a deeper level. Male workers reported that fathers often tend to

Fathers and family centres

identify with them and seek them out; a rapport can be built around 'male' topics of conversation, leading to further 'engagement' with the work of the centre.

> Q: *And do you think having a male member of staff ... makes any difference in terms of getting men involved in the work of the centre?*
>
> *Yeah, I think so. I think they could be relieved when they do see a male here, it does help them. And also ... they can talk about male things in general. Like I have one [father] who's a heavy goods driver and he talks to the males about that because I think he thinks he should be talking about [that] ... I mean I don't know anything about heavy goods driving but you go along with it so to speak, and you can chat with him about that ... And that can lead onto other things ... maybe they do tell you things, you know because you are a male, as well ... they'll say: 'Oh you know what it's like'.*
> (Male worker)

Within men's groups, the gender of the facilitator was regarded as particularly important by fathers.

> Q: *If you were advertising the [men's group], what would you say in your advert to entice people in?*
>
> *'Men's group, run by men. Don't by shy, come in to have a chat.'*
>
> Q: *Why is it important to have a man running it?*
>
> *I think the men are reluctant to talk [to a woman] ... there's certain things that you cannot feel comfortable talking to a woman [about] ... Men's things ... the men's wives, the way you see a woman, relationships and things.*
> (Victor, involved father)

As one mother summed up the debate:

> Q: *Do you think it would make a difference to getting fathers in, if there were more men working in places like this?*
>
> *Yeah, I think there should be a male around. I don't think it would really change the dad ... But I think it would be nice to have a couple of men knocking about. You know it sort of gives the mother-and-dad feel then doesn't it? Because that's what it's all meant to be about isn't it, the family? ... It just gives it that dead warm family feel.*
> (Kelly, mother, uninvolved partner)

Perhaps significantly, none of the 'agnostic' centres had any male presence on the staff and, aside from referred fathers (many of whom nevertheless described themselves as being quite comfortable with women workers), were unlikely to have significant numbers of men present in the centre. Those centres in our sample which did have men as permanent members of staff at the time of the research were all 'gender-blind' in orientation, tending to work with men on what they described as an equal footing to women. Male workers tended to be regarded as useful in these centres, both in providing an initial point of contact in welcoming fathers and as a role model for working with young children (although we found no evidence that the latter served to encourage fathers themselves to engage more fully with the child-oriented activities at the centre). None of those centres with a gender-differentiated approach had male workers. However, their men's groups – where present – were facilitated by male sessional workers, suggesting a degree of role-differentiation at staff, as well as client level.

Enabling factors in men's use of family centres

'People want to do things instead of just sitting around yakking all day' – activity and activities within the family centre

We discussed in the previous chapter how fathers bemoaned the lack of physical activity in family centres, as well as the gendered nature of the (largely sedentary) activities on offer. Even where there were dedicated activities for men, these usually took the form of men's discussion groups and, as we showed, not all men respond well to these. Few centres provided activities specifically targeted at men other than men's groups, therefore we can only speculate about the extent to which different sorts of activities might enable men to become more involved. However, judging from the findings presented in the previous chapter and those reported below, the provision of specific activities for men within family centres, and indeed 'activity' in general, would appear to be a crucial factor in attracting and engaging more men.

For example, barbecues, parties and other types of social, family-oriented events were considered successful in drawing men in:

Like we have special events, you know, one-off events. We had a barbecue. We had loads of fathers who came [to that] *and people knew each other, so* [they] *made groups and they were chatting and all that and the children were playing.*
(Female worker)

When the Christmas party's on up here, fathers come ... there's even uncles that come, and male relatives.
(Terri, mother, uninvolved partner)

This father, who was now uninvolved with the centre, had previously taken part in trips out organised by the family centre and had loved them:

You get the days out like the coach trip to [amusement park]. And it's brilliant. You can get a miniature train that takes you to it and everything. It's pretty good ... for the people who are unemployed. It's not too expensive. [And] *it works better because you're going in a group ... Going in a coach trip rather than just a car – it's nice.*
(Joe, uninvolved father)

Most of the fathers in the sample expressed a desire to have something specific to 'do' at the centre. Such activity could take a number of forms, for example physical play, outings and trips, helping out around the centre; the important thing was to get away from the perceived passivity of the typical family centre 'drop-in', or not be 'stuck in two rooms' as one father put it.

Where men were present in any numbers at a centre, they were generally there with a specific objective in mind. For referred fathers this was implicit – they were involved in a structured programme of work. Casual male visitors to open-access facilities were however rare:

If they've got a course what they're coming to then they've got no problem at all, they'll come straight in because they're coming in for a reason, but if you try to get men just to call in for a cuppa, to have a look round the centre ... You've got no hope.
(Aidan, involved father)

Men often expressed a preference for physical or sporting activities. Occasionally family centres were already running these, but – ironically – preventing men from joining in. For example, this father described with some feeling how disappointed he had been to be prevented

37

Fathers and family centres

from joining in an 'outward bound' type trip because it had been restricted to women only:

Well the girls ... they did a ... thing out on the moor a couple of times. If they had something like that for dads, I wouldn't have minded going along on it. I'm more of an outdoor type than an indoor type.

Q: And you couldn't go on the one with the women?

No, that was taboo that one – for women only.

Q: And you would have (liked to) have done that?

Well yeah, most definitely because I know that place [the moor] like the back of my hand. We'd have had a nice day out. Took some sarnies. Maybe a pot of coffee, something like that. Had a good walk ... or if they'd gone out in a boat for a day or something like that, or ... gone along the river with the kids. I would have done that.
(Frederick, father, no longer involved)

As one worker with experience of running men's activities put it:

Again a lot of the stuff that's worked best within this group functions very much around the focus of [the] 'doing' side, so for instance ... we went on a team-building session at an outdoor pursuit centre and all the guys thought that was really, really good.
(Male worker)

'If there's something that wants fixing ... ' – the desire for a 'masculine' role

Other types of activity mentioned frequently (and even wistfully) by men, when asked to speculate upon how the centre could be improved or made more attractive to men, were practical in nature – such as woodwork, car maintenance, or DIY. We found ample evidence to suggest that men who have some motivation to be involved with the family centre, but are unable to access any appropriate, appealing activity, will create a (suitably masculine) role for themselves. Practical activities, like fixing things around the centre, were especially popular with fathers.

A lot of the men that we did have coming in – if something needed doing, and this is stereotyping again, but you know if something needed fixing or a screw needed [tightening], they would bend over backward to do it.

Q: Why do you think they were so keen to do that?

I don't know. Maybe just 'I'm a man, that's my role, so I'll do it'.

Q: So that suggests that they were keen to get involved?

In something practical, of that nature, yeah, yeah they would.
(Female worker)

I've tried to ... get involved in what's been going on here ... I put a patio down for them ... because the outside was all muddy, and I put some slabs down for them.

Q: Why you?

I offered.
(Graham, involved father)

Q: Can you think of examples when you have changed things or set things up specifically to accommodate men's wishes ... ?

I know we've had men in the past and they've been sat around like twiddling their thumbs, and we've got them to do like maintenance things around the centre, you know a bit of mending,

Enabling factors in men's use of family centres

which has always gone down well really with the men that we've had.
(Female worker)

Staff often felt a little uncomfortable about the stereotyping implied by letting men do these sorts of things. For example, this worker described an ambivalence about allowing men to adopt this role, revealing some (unresolved) contradiction between the workers' and fathers' perceptions of what men should actually be doing whilst in the centre:

We asked [the men] what they would like [if we had a group] and they said, well they want to come, [but] they want to be doing things. But it's very difficult, I mean they helped us put up a cupboard and they've helped us with various things but [just] because they're men you don't want to use them and say, 'Oh look, could you do this and could you do that?'. And then they offered to convert our garage ... but we didn't feel that was their role really ... that wasn't what they were here for.
(Female worker)

But one male worker thought, for men, a focus on 'doing' things was appropriate, because this was how men often defined themselves:

Well, one of the things that's very clear to me is that ... this group of men are very much focused in on doing. [There's a] distinction between a human 'being' and a human 'doing'. But quite often men define themselves by what [they] do ...
(Male worker)

The desire of men to engage in 'meaningful' masculine activity appears to be fundamental, overriding most individual centre-level arrangements. We found examples of men carving out a role for themselves as 'handyman' or general helper in all types of centres, regardless of whether there were any other activities (such as a men's group) aimed at, or of particular interest to, fathers. The level of staff encouragement for such activity varied from ambivalence to active initiation. The most active debate on the pros and cons of allowing, or endorsing, this type of role was encountered in gender-differentiated centres (i.e those already inclined towards a 'men as different' approach).

'I get encouragement' – men's groups within a family centre setting

As we indicated in Chapter 3, the issue of whether the provision of a men's group is in itself an enabling factor is complex. Again, this is an area that would benefit from further study. However, we did find evidence that, for some men at least, men's groups are regarded as empowering and valuable. Men's (or fathers') groups attached to family centres had particular appeal for fathers in exceptional circumstances: lone parents, main carers and non-resident fathers. The primary appeal to these fathers was the opportunity to meet and share experiences with others in similar situations.

What about the contact that you have with other men here? What do you get out of that?

I think I get encouragement. I sort of compare myself with others – situations that they're in, and ... feel much better that I'm not as bad as some others.
(Victor, involved father)

This lone father, whose initial motivation for attending a men's group time was boredom, was palpably relieved and surprised to discover that he was not alone in his predicament.

> *I did have a lot of doubts coming here, I mean the only reason I come in here was because I was bored ... I wasn't looking forward to it at all. But once I sat down and ... the first bloke told me his name, told me how long he'd been a single parent and what problems that he had, [I thought] 'Hey, that's me talking that is' ... I mean that bloke knows why I'm sitting here because that's the reason he's sitting there. And then the next bloke and the next bloke [said the same] ... and I'm [feeling] 'Oh, I'm not on my own. I'm not sitting on a desert island shouting out [all alone]'. There are ... a lot of single fathers who are out there.*
> (Roy, involved father)

The talking done at men's groups was seen by the participants as different from the general feminised 'chat' of the drop-in, or the stereotypical men's conversation about football and sex in the pub. There was something specific that the group could provide for them: support, empathy and advice, within a venue where it was acceptable to be discussing immediate practical issues related to children and parenting.

As we have seen, though, men's groups are by no means appealing to all fathers. Equally, in order to maintain their appeal even to fathers in unusual circumstances, ultimately they need to offer more than a talking shop. Members of men's groups also want to get out and do things on occasion.

One father expressed dissatisfaction with the current inactivity within the group he attended:

> *It's actually drifting apart at the minute because everybody just comes and chats and nothing's actually getting done. So that's why we're looking at doing the bike ride and trying to get more people in ... because people want to do things instead of just sitting around yakking all day.*
> (Jack, involved father)

Related to this, men appreciated it when groups catered to fathers both as men and as parents:

> *When we're off on activities ourselves without the children, it's like a boys' group sometimes really ... like a bunch of lads out ... [but] I mean you have to have a certain element of that anyway. [Because] it's always damn hard work looking after kids ... and it's good to have the group ... to be friends and go out and let off a bit of steam and just have a laugh ... And it's more positive doing it in this group than it is going out and drinking and stuff like that ... And then, the other part of being in the dads' group is being involved with everything else, being involved with the activities involving the kids and all sorts.*
> (Lenny, involved father)

Men's groups were the only types of activity we found which were aimed specifically at fathers in family centres and were all located in centres with a gender-differentiated orientation to working with men. As we have seen, men's groups tended to be attractive to men in particular circumstances (such as lone parents and main carers). It seems that such individual circumstances represent more of a significant enabling factor than the provision of a group *per se*: we found fathers in 'unusual' circumstances seeking out family centres which did not have a men's group, but rarely found 'ordinary' fathers within such groups.

Family centre atmosphere and 'feel'

Finally, we explored the significance of enabling factors connected with the atmosphere or 'feel' of family centres. This was perhaps the most significant barrier identified in Chapter 3, where the feminised environment of family centres was stressed. However, a warm welcome and a relaxing atmosphere could make fathers feel both comfortable and that they belonged, despite being in a minority. The visible presence of other men around the centre was also an advantage.

'You cannot help but want to come back' – feeling welcome

Where family centres succeeded in making men feel accepted, welcomed and valued as a parent, this could, to some extent, counteract the intimidating effects of a female-dominated atmosphere. Some involved fathers described this:

> Q: *What do you particularly like about this place?*
>
> *It's got everything you need ... you come in, you're welcomed, they make you feel welcome, they don't make you an outsider or anything.*
> (Craig, involved father)

> *It is predominantly a female environment ... I stuck out like a sore thumb I suppose ... but the way that I was welcomed by them was ... very, very supportive, it wasn't judgemental that a mother should be doing this or a father's role should be this, it was like 'Come in!'.*
> (Graham, involved father)

More than just an initial ice-breaker, this could set the tone for future visits:

> *I think with this centre ... the staff are so friendly and so welcoming. The volunteers are the same and also the mothers, everybody's just so warm. When you come in the door you cannot help but want to come back.*
> (Lenny, involved father)

Centres that were perceived as having a relaxed atmosphere, and as being helpful and supportive, were also seen as enabling by fathers.

> Q: *And so, when you did come here, what was the impression you got? What kind of place did it feel like?*
>
> *Warm, friendly ... They didn't want to interfere but they want to help you.*
> (Eric, involved father)

'There is a change when you get two men together' – the presence of other men

Arguably, even more important as a way of counteracting the feminised feel of many family centres was the presence of other male users. Men actively sought each other out in heavily female-dominated centres. For example:

> *Yeah, we had one [father] that started [here], he opened up to me and he was telling me this, that and the other and how he was coping with his family and his wife ... There was a lot of things he used to ask me ... I suppose it was because I'm a dad myself, so I suppose he felt a bit more comfortable talking to me.*
> (Derek, involved father)

> Q: *Do you feel you have less in common with women you don't know than men you don't know?*
>
> *Of course you do, of course you do. It's much easier to approach a man that you don't know than a woman ...*
> (Victor, involved father)

Staff had noticed that men together interacted in a more relaxed way:

> *Like the cooking, that's always quite popular with the men and it's nice to see when you get a*

Fathers and family centres

couple of men together in the kitchen, they work totally differently together than they do with the women around ... There is a change when you get two men together.

Q: *What's the difference, what happens?*

Well, they laugh and joke together, and you know they'll joke about ... the women in their lives and things that are going on, and they talk about employment and they talk about the past, and they talk about mutual interests. Not very many men do that I've found, when they're on their own [in here].

Q: *They don't talk like that with the women?*

No, not very often. It's a different kind of relationship.
(Female worker)

Why did men feel so much more relaxed around other men? One reason may be, as some fathers suggested, that women see themselves as child-care 'experts' and could be somewhat dismissive about men's struggles with child rearing. Men, on the other hand, were more likely to help boost each other's self-esteem:

If [something has happened, for example] *like I say 'Jeeze, my kid shit herself all over, and I've had to clean it all up. Oh God'* [with] *a bloke, you can make a laugh out of it, have a joke, but if you tell a woman she'd say 'So what, I do that anyway', short and sharp.* [Whereas] *if you tell a bloke, you get a bit of praise, you get: 'Oh God, man, I couldn't do that'.*
(Phil, involved father)

As we stated earlier, there was some male presence in every centre visited, and our 'involved' fathers described being made to feel welcome and included by staff in a variety of different settings and circumstances. However, as we have seen already, these 'involved' fathers had often been initially motivated to attend the centre by some 'higher-order' enabler (such as referral, or particular circumstances). A welcoming atmosphere, or indeed the presence of other men, thus appears to serve more as a bonus – and as an incentive to revisit – than as an entry-level factor.

5 Conclusions and implications for policy and practice

The evidence from this study is that a lot of what keeps fathers out of family centres is related to the way family centres are seen and experienced – by fathers, mothers and staff alike – as 'women's places' or as 'women-and-children's places'. In the current social climate, despite increasing debate and changing social attitudes and expectations in the sphere of family life, women continue to be seen as – and indeed generally are – the main carers of the nation's children. As our data clearly show, family-support services, like family centres, are therefore not always seen as relevant to fathers, except to those who are 'unusual' in some way – perhaps in special circumstances (e.g. lone fathers, fathers who are main carers whilst mothers work, fathers from families in difficulties who are referred for therapeutic work), or perhaps with 'special' and unusual levels of attachment and commitment to family activities. These groups are almost certainly increasing in size (Burghes *et al.*, 1997), and the signs are that they will keep growing well. Encouragingly, family centres already successfully cater to these groups to some extent and can probably continue to meet at least some of the needs of these fathers, with relatively little change to current structure and functioning.

While focusing on the increasing diversity in family structures and arrangements within the UK, it is important not to forget that most children still grow up within intact, two-parent, first-time families. Even within the disadvantaged communities that family centres typically serve, most fathers are not lone parents, main carers, or from families with problems requiring therapeutic intervention. Moreover, it is probably true that highly involved and committed fathers are also still a minority group amongst fathers in general. The picture for family centres which want to attract in these 'ordinary' fathers looks a little more challenging.

Who are family centres for? – 'child-focused' versus 'family-focused' services

This study revealed a complex network of barriers and enabling factors which work to prevent and promote fathers' use of family centres. Some of these factors were rooted in broad social and cultural attitudes. Others appeared to be intricately bound up with individual men's family, relationship and personal circumstances. Yet the most frequently mentioned incentives and disincentives to family centre use were not located at the cultural or personal level, but at the institutional one, and could be clearly traced back to the way in which family centres are structured, managed, staffed and organised. As we tried to disentangle the reasons for this, we found ourselves asking a very basic question: who and what are family centres for?

It is clear that centres are fundamentally for children and that much of what they do is carried out with the intention of enhancing children's well-being across a range of dimensions. What is less clear is the role of adult users within family centres. For example, are adult users viewed only as parents or carers of children and seen as having needs only in relation to their children's needs? If so, this would suggest that family centres are best described as *child-focused*: children come first, and parents come along as part of the package. Under this definition, centres would structure

Fathers and family centres

priorities and activities mainly around child-care and enhancing specific parenting skills (for example, using play activities and parent education). On the other hand, some centres would say that they also try to cater to parents as adults in their own right, recognising parents' separate, and sometimes different, needs from children. The underlying rationale for such an approach would be that enhancing parents' confidence and empowering them to function better in general would be expected to have indirect benefits in terms of more confident parenting and better parent–child relationships. In this case, we might define centres as *family-focused*, and we would expect to find a range of activities taking place, some of which were perhaps only tangentially related to child-care (for example, adult education).

What we found in this study was that most centres are, in fact, a mixture of child-focused and family-focused in their approach, and that the type of approach is mediated by the sex of the user. Often, family centres are family-focused in their approach to working with women and child-focused in their approach to working with men. So, for example, where women were concerned, there seemed to be no unease about letting mothers relate to family centres as women, as well as mothers. Indeed, this was positively encouraged in most family centres, where the philosophy that happy, fulfilled and empowered women make better mothers is translated into a wide range of activities that do not always involve, or revolve around, children. When talking about the mothers who used the centre, staff stressed the importance of accepting women 'on their own terms', being non-judgemental, and providing skills-related and creative or therapeutic activities that arose out of women's own agendas and were designed to enhance self-esteem. That this was a successful approach was reflected in our study (as in others – e.g. Smith, 1996; Pithouse and Holland, 1999) by the positive perceptions of women users about the value and impact of the centre on their lives.

Yet, where fathers were concerned, a rather different set of priorities appeared to arise. Our data suggested that some centres seemed to experience a level of unease about allowing men in 'on their own terms', in an equivalent way to women users. Indeed, it sometimes seemed that men were welcome in family centres as fathers, but not as men in their own right, whereas women were welcomed as mothers and women both. Thus, few centres offered or encouraged the development of any activities of interest or appeal to men that did not revolve directly around child-care. Men were rarely given the opportunity of participating in what they defined as 'men's activities', as opposed to 'children's activities' or 'women's activities'. As a result, there were difficulties in engaging men's interest in family centres, beyond seeing them as simply places of play for their children. Furthermore, though this function as a child's play-space was certainly appreciated by fathers, men often talked about feeling unable to relax and 'be themselves' (that is, be men) whilst at centres. Tellingly, whenever the opportunity arose, it seemed fathers in family centres tried to subvert the role planned for them and create a more 'manly' or 'masculine' role for themselves – usually by making themselves physically useful. And, although this was often a route into feeling more 'legitimate' as a man within a family centre, it was frequently regarded with ambivalence by centre staff. Finally, some

Conclusions and implications for policy and practice

centres had tried to create a separate space for men (for example, by setting up a men's group) but these tended to be almost ghettoised and were certainly rather marginal to the work of the centre as a whole. Indeed, the data suggested that men who wanted successfully to engage with the full range of family centre activities were often only able to do so if they were prepared to come on women's terms and, more or less, become pseudo-women. Not surprisingly, not all fathers relish becoming 'one of the girls' (as one father put it) and many men voted with their feet.

The need for clarity of focus

The foregoing suggests that there is a pressing need for clarity in policy and service planning, in respect of how best to engage fathers in family-support services. We began this research on the assumption that family centres, occupying as they do a position at the heart of mainstream services for children, ought to be considered as appropriate services from which to engage with fathers. Many would share this assumption: our study revealed that there is increasing interest amongst family centre practitioners in engaging with fathers and there are already some well-known examples of successful practice in this area, for example, Pen Green Family Centre (Ghedini *et al.*, 1995). However, our findings led us to question whether this assumption necessarily holds true for all, or even many, centres.

If family centres continue to approach work with fathers as they presently do, from a mainly child-focused perspective, our data suggested that there are probably relatively few men to whom family centres will appeal. Unlike women, they will find little to engage their attention as adults, rather than just as parents, and centres are therefore likely to remain female-dominated and women-focused. As a result, there will continue to be too few men using any given centre to attain the 'critical mass' situation that would, according to our findings, make men feel more comfortable. The only men who will use such centres on a regular basis will continue to be, as now, those in unusual circumstances, those who have been directed to attend, or those who are seen as being somewhat 'different' from most men. The majority of fathers will continue, as now, to feel alienated and excluded.

Similar observations led one recent study to query, on the basis of research in two open-access family centres:

Can family centres really claim to be dealing with the 'family'? ... If centres are gender-biased and attract narrow ranges of ... users then there is good reason to question whether such places work with families in any clear sense and whether the term 'family centre' summarises most aptly the function of the setting.
(Pithouse and Holland, 1999, p. 173)

One worker in our sample took this idea a little further:

Men don't traditionally meet in a family centre, for various reasons, and so [in] *trying to change things here, perhaps we're trying to create something artificial? Would our efforts not be best spent ... actually going to where the men are ...* [where they] *feel comfortable in the first place?*
(Male worker)

Fathers and family centres

This worker seems to be suggesting that service provision for fathers may have to be revisited. Perhaps rather than 'tacking on' services for fathers to those which already work for women, but may not be easily adapted to men's needs, we need to consider establishing whole new 'father-support' services, designed and structured with fathers in mind. There is evidence that this is already happening in some areas and it may be that new services have a better chance of success in this field.

However, many would feel that family centres could and should be able to cater to fathers, as well as mothers. New services are expensive to set up, and building on existing service networks is likely to be more cost-effective in the short to medium term. As Pithouse and Holland (1999) venture, ('heretically', they admit), perhaps it is just not enough to 'justify the costs of this type of preventive service' to say that family centres work well to satisfy adult female users. If male users are not catered to, can centres really be said to be optimally effective in a family-support context? Furthermore, is there not a risk that calling such a service a 'family centre' and then failing to cater to parents of both sexes could unwittingly reinforce gender stereotypes, in relation to child care and 'proper' roles within the family?

No doubt this is an issue that could be debated far more extensively and widely than we are able to do here. However, on the basis of the findings from this study, our view is that, if it is considered appropriate to try to engage with fathers, then at least some of the existing national network of family centres might well prove ideal for this purpose. First, however, we need to consider how centres can do this and be turned into places which cater better to men and make them feel accepted on their own terms – as men, as well as fathers. Our research suggested a number of ways in which men could be enabled to use family centres, through – to use our term – a 'family-focused' model of work, but some of these might involve centres in a substantial shift in terms of approach and atmosphere. We discuss this below.

Making family centres father-friendly: possible directions for change in policy and practice

The first and most important change necessary would be to reduce the level of female dominance within family centres. Centres would need to encourage more positive, accepting and actively welcoming attitudes towards men in women users and staff and, in particular, discourage women from giving vent to the kind of anti-male sentiments that were illustrated in Chapter 3 of this report. *Not all centres would regard this as a route that they would want to travel.* Precisely because they are women-dominated, family centres are often places of 'refuge' for many vulnerable women – places to get away from unsatisfactory and damaging relationships. For others, centres are places to feel relaxed, supported and powerful in ways not possible at home or elsewhere. As Burgess and Ruxton (1996) put it: 'A concern for many female staff and service users is that increasing male involvement may displace them from one of the few arenas … in which they are able to exert power over their lives'. Some centres may be able comfortably to accommodate both women and men in separate spaces, or at different times, but not all will have

Conclusions and implications for policy and practice

the resources necessary for this, even if they have the inclination.

The second area for change would be a positive commitment on the part of centres to recruit men, backed up by action – and persistent action at that. As we have shown in Chapter 4, personal introductions, where staff actively seek out potential male users and persuade them into the centre, are important for overcoming the various barriers to fathers' reticence and nervousness. Persistence appears to be required, with some men having to be asked 'hundreds' of times before they pay the centre a visit. This, of course, requires resources as well as commitment. 'Pyramid selling' also needs to be actively encouraged, according to our respondents – getting existing users to invite potential new recruits. Women's encouragement of their partners is important in this respect, but the best salesmen are likely to be existing male users.

Third, better promotion of the centre's activities was mentioned as an area for improvement by many of our respondents and especially by uninvolved men. Many had only a sketchy idea of what went on in the centre and accurate information might dispel some of the perceptions of men about activities consisting solely of gossip and focusing on 'women's problems'. Some men pointed out that even the names of centres tended to mislead potential male users, feeling that the very words 'family' and 'parents' were so female-identified that not all fathers would recognise themselves as included in the target clientele. The need to announce to passing men that fathers' participation was also welcome was pressing, as this uninvolved father pointed out:

I think a lot of men probably just don't really know what it's about. [They] *need to make it quite clear that both parents are welcome. When you hear the word parent, somehow you link it with the mother more. You tend to forget that* [a family centre] *is actually a place where both parents can be.*
(Hassan, uninvolved father)

Fourthly and finally, if fathers are to be encouraged into family centres in sufficient numbers to reach the critical mass that will make them feel comfortable, a different approach to providing activities is almost certainly required. By this, we mean both activities that men will find interesting and meaningful, and 'activity' in the physical sense of the word. By and large, most fathers do not find the activities that currently characterise family centres very stimulating. Active play with children was welcomed (*kicking a ball around* and playing *on the bikes* or *in the sandpit* were mentioned by several men), but fathers often found the quiet play, 'child watching', arts and crafts, and health and beauty sessions, which are the staple of many centres, boring and, in the case of the last two, sometimes downright 'unmanly'. 'Sitting and chatting' to other parents was also, in general, not seen as very productive by men. On the basis of this study, it seems likely that what might attract greater numbers of fathers to family centres would be outdoor and sport-related activities, excursions and trips, and productive, skills-related activities, such as DIY, computer skills and other adult-education activities.

Related to this, the question of dedicated men's groups and whether they are a pre-requisite for engaging with fathers is one we

Fathers and family centres

struggled with. Men who were members of groups valued them; of that there is no doubt. However, many groups were infrequently attended, and seemed very much on the periphery of the centre. Some were almost completely autonomous and hardly part of the rest of the family centre at all. Most of the men who attended had taken a great deal of persuasion to get involved and all bemoaned the fact that it was hard to recruit new members. As we showed earlier, non-users had ambivalent, if not actually negative, views of the groups. We concluded, therefore, that, although men's groups are enabling for some, they may not be a first-line of service provision. Providing a men's group alone is unlikely to be a successful way to recruit large numbers of fathers. Rather, men's groups should perhaps be viewed as an 'advanced' activity for established users of centres.

Perhaps some of the ambivalence we picked up amongst family centre staff about encouraging 'men's' activities reflected a worry that allowing men to pursue alternative activities might lead them away from their children, rather than enhancing their parenting skills and relationships with children:

> *If you put too much men interest into it for the fathers, then they will be off doing that, and not take any notice of the kids.*
> (Neil, uninvolved father)

However, in the USA, a good practice guide to working with men makes the point that a strategic approach to involving fathers which enhances the interest for them as men, not just fathers, is likely, in the long run, to be more effective:

> *One of the best ways to get men more involved with their children and your program is to not ask them to get more involved with their children and your program. The explanation for that puzzling contradiction is actually quite simple. Before they can take care of their children's needs, all parents need to feel that someone is helping take care of their needs ... For many men, the most comfortable way to get involved is through activities that they think of as 'men's work' – fixing things ... So, one of the best ways to get men hooked into your program is by helping them to connect with other men in 'manly' ways. Once they have other guys to relate to in your program they may feel more comfortable about participating with children.*
> (Levine et al. 1993, pp. 37–8)

Or, as this father put it:

> *It has to be a playing environment where you can take notice of the kids, but still have something to occupy your mind.*
> (Neil, uninvolved father)

To conclude, parenting is not a gender-neutral activity. Though mothering and fathering share a common core of skills, men and women have different things to contribute to their children, and often have different approaches to parenting. The challenge for family centres that want to cater to parents of both sexes (and some, very possibly, will *not* want to do this) is to enable both women and men to access and use the service in ways that recognise diversity, and which play to men and women's different strengths and interests. There is probably no one right way to do this and our concept of centre orientation is helpful here. It is clear that, at a basic level, having a strategy and a commitment to involving men is more

Conclusions and implications for policy and practice

important than what precise approach is taken to achieve this. Thus both 'gender-blind' and 'gender-differentiated' centres in our study were doing better at getting men engaged at entry level than 'agnostic' ones. At a deeper level, however, centres wishing to cater to fathers may find that listening to what local men say they want, and being prepared to try fresh approaches to providing and facilitating activities, may be the most effective way to achieving what is truly a 'family' centre.

References

Burgess, A. and Ruxton, S. (1996) *Men and their Children: Proposals for Public Policy.* London: IPPR

Burghes, L., Clarke, L. and Cronin, N. (1997) *Fathers and Fatherhood in Britain.* London: Family Policy Studies Centre

Ghate, D., Shaw, C. and Hazel, N. (2000) *Fathers at the Centre: Family Centres, Fathers and Working with Men.* Internet Publication at: http://www.rip.co.uk/rep/fathers/index.html

Ghedini, P., Chandler, T., Whalley, M. and Moss, P. (1995) *Fathers, Nurseries and Child Care.* European Commission Network on Childcare

Glaser, B.G. and Straus, A.L. (1967) *The Discovery of Grounded Theory.* Chicago: Aldine

Kraemer, S. (1995) 'What are fathers for?', in C. Burke and B. Speed (eds) *Gender, Power and Relationships.* London: Routledge

Kuckartz, U. (1998) WinMax Pro (software program) available from Scolari Sage Publications Software

Lamb, M. (1996) *The Role of the Father in Child Development.* Chichester: John Wiley

Levine, J.A. and Pitt, E.W. (1995) *New Expectations: Community Strategies for Responsible Fatherhood.* New York: Families and Work Institute

Levine, J.A., Murphy, D.T. and Wilson, S. (1993) *Getting Men Involved: Strategies for Early Childhood Programs.* New York: Scholastic

Pithouse, A. and Holland, S. (1999) 'Open access family centres and their users: positive results, some doubts and new departures', *Children and Society,* Vol. 13, No. 3, pp. 167–78

Pugh, G. (1992) 'A policy for early childhood services', in G. Pugh (ed.) *Contemporary Issues in the Early Years.* London: Chapman

Pugh, G., De'Ath, E. and Smith, C. (1994) *Confident Parents, Confident Children: Policy and Practice in Parent Education and Support.* London: National Children's Bureau

Ritchie, J. and Spencer, L. (1994) 'Qualitative data analysis for applied policy research', in A. Bryman and R.G Burgess (eds) *Analyzing qualitative data.* London: Routledge

Smith, T. (1996) *Family Centres and Looking After Young Children.* London: HMSO

Appendix 1: Practice issues in engaging with fathers in family centres

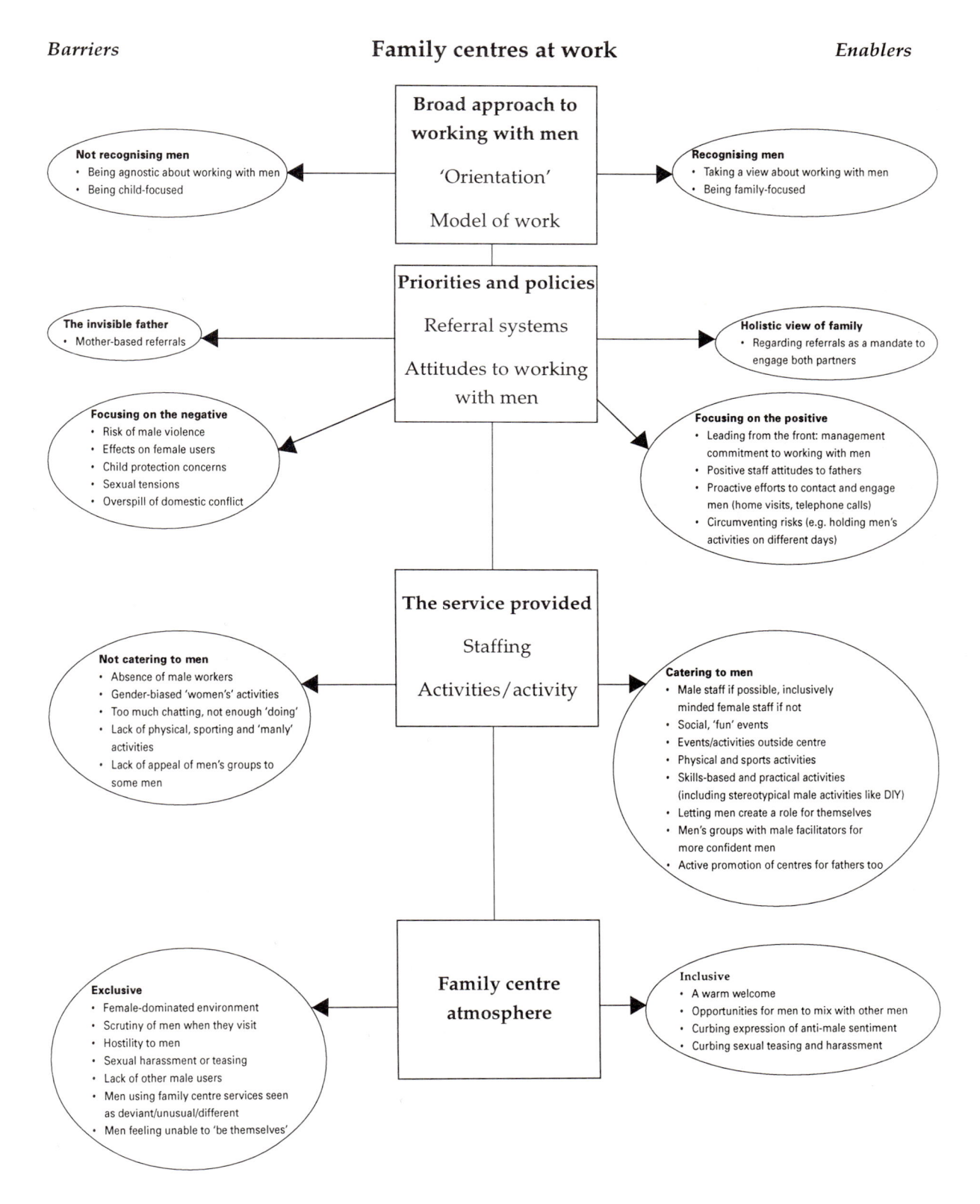

Barriers   Family centres at work   *Enablers*

Broad approach to working with men
'Orientation'
Model of work

- **Not recognising men**
  - Being agnostic about working with men
  - Being child-focused

- **Recognising men**
  - Taking a view about working with men
  - Being family-focused

Priorities and policies
Referral systems
Attitudes to working with men

- **The invisible father**
  - Mother-based referrals

- **Holistic view of family**
  - Regarding referrals as a mandate to engage both partners

- **Focusing on the negative**
  - Risk of male violence
  - Effects on female users
  - Child protection concerns
  - Sexual tensions
  - Overspill of domestic conflict

- **Focusing on the positive**
  - Leading from the front: management commitment to working with men
  - Positive staff attitudes to fathers
  - Proactive efforts to contact and engage men (home visits, telephone calls)
  - Circumventing risks (e.g. holding men's activities on different days)

The service provided
Staffing
Activities/activity

- **Not catering to men**
  - Absence of male workers
  - Gender-biased 'women's' activities
  - Too much chatting, not enough 'doing'
  - Lack of physical, sporting and 'manly' activities
  - Lack of appeal of men's groups to some men

- **Catering to men**
  - Male staff if possible, inclusively minded female staff if not
  - Social, 'fun' events
  - Events/activities outside centre
  - Physical and sports activities
  - Skills-based and practical activities (including stereotypical male activities like DIY)
  - Letting men create a role for themselves
  - Men's groups with male facilitators for more confident men
  - Active promotion of centres for fathers too

Family centre atmosphere

- **Exclusive**
  - Female-dominated environment
  - Scrutiny of men when they visit
  - Hostility to men
  - Sexual harassment or teasing
  - Lack of other male users
  - Men using family centre services seen as deviant/unusual/different
  - Men feeling unable to 'be themselves'

- **Inclusive**
  - A warm welcome
  - Opportunities for men to mix with other men
  - Curbing expression of anti-male sentiment
  - Curbing sexual teasing and harassment

Appendix 2: Range of activities taking place in sample family centres

Activities for pre-school children
Day-care, nursery education, creche, special needs playgroup.

Activities for older children/young people
After-school clubs, school holiday schemes, homework facilities, therapeutic group for young people, young gay/lesbian support group, youth club, teenagers' coffee bar, classes for excluded pupils.

Activities for parents and children together
Playgroups, parent/child literacy programme, 'High Scope' programme, treasure baskets and heuristic play, music workshop, creative/messy play sessions, family art/craft workshops.

Support for individuals and families
Tailored family-support programmes, informal one-to-one support, formal counselling, preparation for adoption (children), family therapy, referral to other agencies.

Adult education
Self-esteem programme, parenting courses, communication skills, creative writing, healthy child project, return to learning, English as an additional language, visiting speakers (health/welfare issues).

Leisure activities for parents (groups)
Keep fit, health/beauty, aromatherapy/massage/relaxation, Tai chi, art and crafts, sewing, machine knitting, flower arranging, cooking, cake decorating, furniture restoration.

Support groups (adult)
Asian women, men, ante-natal, post-natal, post-natal depression, childminder and nanny.

Statutory work
Assessment, supervised contact.

Other facilities and services available to families
Adult/children's library, toy library, drop-in area, office facilities, bath/shower, kitchen and laundry facilities, saving/credit union schemes, second-hand clothing.

External activities
Home visits, in-home support work, outreach sessions in other settings (primary schools, community centres, village halls), mobile centre, trips and outings for parents (e.g. shopping, lunch, theatre, ten-pin bowling), trips and outings for families (e.g. leisure centre, park, farm, seaside).

Access to health professionals (on-site surgery or drop-in)
Health visitor, speech therapist, child psychologist.

Miscellaneous
Food parcels, escorting children to/from contact sessions.

Appendix 3: Pen portraits of family centres

All names of centres have been changed to preserve the anonymity of interviewees.

Green Square Parents' Centre (type B)
Inner London, voluntary sector
Green Square serves the families of a diverse and densely populated area of inner London. The immediate neighbourhood contains a substantial Bengali community and a wide diversity of other ethnic groups, including the families of mature students from overseas and refugees. The centre runs a daily drop-in facility for parents and carers, recreational and educational classes for parents (with creche), plus after-school and holiday provision for older children.

Whilst fathers are actively welcomed, few currently attend on a regular basis. The centre has one male member of staff and has recently prioritised developing its work with fathers.

The Bungalow Family Centre [type E (A + D)]
Inner London, local authority
Situated in a borough with a mixed social and ethnic profile, The Bungalow works exclusively with referred families and children. Most families are referred for assessment purposes and are worked with on an individual basis by social workers (one of whom is male). Supervised contact sessions are also facilitated. The Bungalow also runs a day-care facility to which children may be referred by social workers or health visitors.

Fathers are worked with if present in a referred family; there is little contact with fathers of children attending the nursery.

Hillside Family Centre [type E (B + D)]
Unitary authority (Wales), local authority
Whilst situated on an inner city council estate, Hillside nevertheless serves a wide catchment area. Transport is provided for children referred (mainly by health visitors) to the thrice-weekly day-care sessions and their parents are encouraged to attend the weekly parents' group. Other activities, such as playgroups, after-school clubs, courses and a weekly drop-in, are open to parents from the local community.

Few fathers become involved in the activities on offer.

Valley Cross Family Centre (type C)
Unitary authority (Wales), voluntary sector
Valley Cross Family Centre serves a fairly isolated estate some distance from the city centre, an area of high unemployment and deprivation. Many of the families on the estate are either reconstituted, or headed by lone mothers.

Paid workers support volunteers from the community in setting up and running groups and activities, including a daily playgroup, after-school clubs and holiday play-schemes. There is a coffee bar used by parents during the day and a youth group in the evening. Fathers' involvement in the centre is minimal.

Fathers and family centres

Quayside Family Centre (type A)
Metropolitan borough (North of England), local authority
Quayside Family Centre is situated in a recently redeveloped inner city area which has a predominantly white population. The centre works with referred families only, individual programmes of work being devised according to need. This may include support in the home, as well as centre-based work. Supervised contact also takes place at the centre. Increasingly, the work of the centre revolves around assessments for court, whilst group-work and drop-in provision (for current and ex-users of the centre) has declined.

Fathers are worked with if present in a referred family.

Phoenix Family Centre [type E (A + B)]
Metropolitan borough (North of England), partnership
Phoenix Family Centre serves a relatively insular and established community, located several miles from the city centre. On three days a week, families referred by social services attend structured sessions, mainly for assessment purposes. At other times, the centre is open to the local community, offering classes, a drop-in day facility and after-school facilities for young people.

The centre has two male workers (one full-time, one sessional), and aims to integrate fathers into all aspects of its provision.

Nightingale Family Centre (type A)
City (Midlands), voluntary sector
Based in a community centre, Nightingale Family Centre is currently open for two days a week in order to provide support to mothers of under-fives. Nursery facilities are provided for their children. Mothers are referred to the centre from across the city and transport is available if necessary. The focus is on adult education, which is provided by sessional tutors from the local college.

Following interest expressed by some of the women's partners, funding has recently been raised to start a fathers' group at the centre.

Field Lane Family Centre [type E (D + B)]
City (Midlands), local authority
Situated in an ethnically mixed area close to the city centre, Field Lane is one of several family centres run by the local social services department. While offering a range of services to local families, day-care is the core activity at Field Lane. Both full-time and sessional placements are available for children in need and those with a working lone parent. There is a daily drop-in facility, open to parents from the local community, and a number of groups are run.

Field Lane has a well-established men's group, facilitated by a male sessional worker.

High Street Family Centre (type B)
County (South West), partnership
Situated in the centre of a small, but socially diverse, town and open on four days a week, High Street Family Centre provides a range of open-access activities for parents and under-fives. There is a daily drop-in session, craft and play-oriented groups for parents and children together and some groups just for parents (with creche provision). High Street also has a mobile facility which visits ten isolated communities

each week, offering a similar range of services.

The small number of fathers using the town-based centre rejected the offer of a separate fathers' group. In one village visited by the mobile facility, equal numbers of fathers and mothers became involved, although elsewhere the outreach service catered primarily to mothers.

White Lodge Family Centre (type A)
County (South West), local authority
White Lodge Family Centre serves a large geographical area, providing transport for those families who attend the centre. In addition to centre-based staff there is a team of community-based family support workers. All referrals come via social services and individual programmes of work are devised and reviewed on a three-monthly basis. Most of the centre-based work is carried out on an individual basis, although occasionally groups are provided according to need. There is a staffed play room for children.

The manager of the centre is the only male member of staff. Fathers are worked with when part of a referred family.

River View Early Years Centre [type D (with B)]
City (North of England), local authority
River View Early Years Centre was formed when a family centre and a nursery school were merged on a single, newly furbished site close to the city centre. Most of the centre users come from the immediate neighbourhood, which is one of high deprivation, but others travel from more affluent areas to use the nursery provision. Full-time nursery places are available in the nursery for two to five year olds. Parents are encouraged to stay in the family room with the younger children. In addition, the centre offers after-school and holiday provision for older children and courses for parents.

Lots of fathers drop off and pick up their children from the nursery, but fewer participate in the other activities at the centre.

Flatlands Children and Families Project [type B (with C)]
County (East Anglia), voluntary sector
Flatlands, while based on a housing estate in a small town, also serves the wider community through outreach work in isolated villages and local schools. It offers a range of services, including support-groups, play activities, after-school and holiday provision for children and young people. Users may be referred by social services, although most are self-referrals. The project does not undertake statutory assessment work.

There is a small self-run men's group, set up by a local father, which meets weekly at the project.

Brownfield fathers' group [type E (B + C) centre]
City (North of England), partnership
Brownfield fathers' group had been in existence for less than a year at the time of the interviews. It had been initiated as a central feature of a newly established family centre, serving a deprived inner city area with a predominantly white population.

The fathers' group, consisting of about six core members and facilitated by a male sessional worker, meets weekly. The group is

Fathers and family centres

open to all fathers in the area and includes fathers with a range of family circumstances, including lone parenthood, non-residence and those in reconstituted families.